FOR WEIGHT LOSS THAT'S RAPID— AND PERMANENT

"You can lose up to 10% of your total weight in the first 7 days," says Richard Hittleman who has as much experience with obesity problems as any person in the U.S.

Through Yoga, you can lose weight—and inches—and keep that correct weight the rest of your life.
Through a unique program of Yoga Nutrition, natural exercises and optional fasting—you can attain a new beauty, vitality, peace of spirit and self-confidence.
For only Yoga, by changing the way you think about yourself, keeps you thin forever.

After you've read this book,
you may never need to diet again!
TRY these exercises you'll look forward to doing. . .
the dieting without a sense of denial . . . fasting that's not starvation, but actually cleanses
and rebuilds your body.
TRY *Yoga Weight Loss for a total new way of life!*

Bantam Books by Richard Hittleman
Ask your bookseller for the books you have missed

RICHARD HITTLEMAN'S GUIDE TO YOGA
    MEDITATION
RICHARD HITTLEMAN'S INTRODUCTION TO
    YOGA
RICHARD HITTLEMAN'S YOGA 28 DAY
    EXERCISE PLAN
WEIGHT CONTROL THROUGH YOGA
YOGA NATURAL FOODS COOKBOOK

WEIGHT CONTROL THROUGH YOGA

BY
RICHARD HITTLEMAN

BANTAM BOOKS · TORONTO · NEW YORK · LONDON

WEIGHT CONTROL THROUGH YOGA

*A Bantam Book / published by arrangement
with Workman Publishing Company, Inc.*

Bantam edition / June 1971

2nd printing . . . . . . January 1971	7th printing . . . . July 1976
3rd printing . . . . September 1972	8th printing . . . . July 1977
4th printing . . . . May 1973	9th printing . . . . . . January 1978
5th printing . . . . . December 1974	10th printing . . . . . . January 1979
6th printing . . . . May 1975	11th printing . . . . July 1980

ISBN 0-553-14313-1

Published simultaneously in the United States and Canada

*Bantam Books are published by Bantam Books, Inc. Its trade-
mark, consisting of the words "Bantam Books" and the por-
trayal of a bantam, is Registered in U.S. Patent and Trademark
Office and in other countries. Marca Registrada. Bantam
Books, Inc., 666 Fifth Avenue, New York, New York 10019.*

PRINTED IN THE UNITED STATES OF AMERICA

20 19 18 17 16 15 14 13 12 11

CONTENTS

INTRODUCTION

I believe I have had as much experience with the problem of obesity as any person in the United States. My *Yoga for Health* television programs have brought me into contact with tens of thousands of overweight viewers, and through the years I have had the opportunity not only to suggest various applications of the Yoga techniques to the problem of obesity, but to learn directly from these viewers the results they attained.

Here, for the first time in written form, we offer the plan that has been tested the most extensively and found to be the most successful—The Yoga Weight-Loss Plan. This special combination of Yoga exercises and Yoga principles of nutrition results in a dramatic loss of pounds and inches, a significant redistribution of weight, and a rapid firming of flabby areas. It is designed for use by *all* overweight people, regardless of the degree of obesity.

In addition to the plan I've just described, here for the first time, too, is a unique Yoga Fasting Program. "I could never fast," you say. *But fasting is not starving— it is cleansing and rebuilding.* You are offered three fasts —a Partial Fast, a Liquid Fast and a Total Fast. Each is explained—why it works, what it can do for your body (besides weight loss)—and how you can do it, with a full section on your questions and answers. By fasting, you can actually lose up to 10% of your body weight the first seven days, encouraging results that can give you the enthusiasm to continue with the somewhat less spectacular, but eventually life-changing Yoga Weight-Loss Plan.

Here are some of the things this book can do for you:
1. You can lose whatever number of pounds and inches necessary for you.
2. You can maintain your correct weight permanently. No more downs-and-up-agains.
3. The exercises are natural—no strain, no fatigue. They become a part of your life.
4. Yoga exercises give you beauty, strength, vitality, peace of mind.
5. The Life Force (*Prana*) you gain from Hatha Yoga will provide the incentive you need to ensure dieting success.
6. You gain a whole new way of life—with enriched meaning—as well as a new way of eating and exercising.

Use the plan of this book, and you will be able not only to attain—but to maintain your normal weight permanently. Once this has been accomplished, it is my fervent hope that you will not be content to utilize the profound Yoga techniques solely for these purposes—but will be moved to serious consideration of incorporating the total science and philosophy of Yoga into your daily life.

—Richard L. Hittleman
Carmel, California 1971

SECTION ONE

THE
YOGA THEORY
OF
WEIGHT REGULATION

CHAPTER 1

HOW THE YOGA WEIGHT LOSS PLAN DIFFERS FROM ALL OTHERS

There is the story of the man from the city who is spending his annual two-week vacation at a summer resort noted for the excellence and abundance of its cuisine. Since he has chosen the "American Plan" in which three daily meals are included, he feels it is his duty to take full advantage of the arrangement.

Accordingly, he is seen spending the better part of the two weeks in the dining room, voraciously consuming the multitude of tasty dishes set before him and frequently requesting "seconds" of whatever strikes his fancy. In addition, he is always on hand for the mid-morning, mid-afternoon and pre-bedtime snacks. In this manner he is quick to sport an excess of at least ten pounds and knowledgeable observers are· privately commenting that he is a sure bet to make it up to twenty.

One evening at the dinner table, upon finishing his second helping of a chocolate mousse, he stiffens in his chair and with heart pounding and blood pressure racing upward, falls to the floor in a dead faint. The waiter, seeing what has happened, races to him with a glass of water and forces a few drops through his colorless lips. Slowly the man regains consciousness. One eyelid flickers and is slowly raised. Looking down at the hand of the waiter he gasps in a hoarse whisper, "Water? Who ordered water? Bring me a milk shake!"

The absurd overindulgence of this man makes us laugh. And yet, an ever-increasing number of overweight Americans, while usually requiring a period of more than two weeks, are committing a similar type of suicide. The statistics are staggering; overweight has become a national joke and a national tragedy. As a result there are thousands of dissertations available on the subject of weight loss. Formerly fat psychiatrists, thin joggers, muscular Air Force men, aging movie starlets, Japanese vegetarians, drinking men, numerous food packagers and those never-ending sources of "miracle" plans—magazines and Sunday supplements—are but a few of the popular contributors to weight-control literature.

A vast new industry has emerged, merchandising an infinite number of "slenderizing" products that include pull, push and peddle apparatuses, friction machines, appetite deterrents in the form of pills, powders and wafers, liquid diets, heat and steam contraptions and, if all else fails, various garments that will, at least, make people *think* you're thinner. In addition there are all grades of salons and spas where inches and pounds are magically "melted" away (and magically return) as well as "weight clubs," cropping up everywhere, which offer a type of group non-eating therapy. With all these machines, clubs, salons and diet aids as well as such voluminous exercising and diet literature available to the overweight person, why *another* book—even a Yoga book—on the subject of weight loss? Hasn't it all been said?

Inherent in the system of Yoga is a physical and philosophical approach to the weight problem, to exercise and diet, that is totally different from the concepts that are currently being offered to the overweight public. Contact with thousands of overweight people has allowed me to observe that very few, if any, of the weight-control devices, gadgets and plans have proven truly satisfactory, *especially in the long run*. I attribute this failure primarily to the fact that, with very few exceptions, the approaches to the problem of obesity are fragmented. The overweight person is being advised to *superimpose* various diet and exercise plans on his life—plans that are generally very much out of context with the type of life he is leading. The attempt to incorporate them into daily activities feels forced and unnatural; consequently, they meet with only temporary or partial success or they fail entirely.

11

If weight control takes the form of a perpetual battle, a never-ending intrusion wherein the "good you" must keep a constant vigil lest the "bad you" indulge in weight-gaining activities, life becomes complicated and uncomfortable. In the long view it is unrealistic for the overweight person to seek a special solution to obesity, that is, to isolate it as a particular problem apart from his *total pattern* of living. *Permanent regulation and control of weight must be natural by-products of the total way in which one lives!*

Instead of attempting to graft various plans for weight control onto an existing mode of life, the most practical and successful solution to the problem is to alter the *way of life*. It is possible to undertake a manner of living in which weight regulation and permanent control are inevitable; wherein, among many other positive things, "exercising" is looked forward to as one of the most enjoyable activities of the day and "dieting" harbors no sense of denial or restriction. Yoga is just such a total way of life. In accordance with this overall concept of changing the basic patterns of living, here is how the material of this particular book applies specifically to the immediate problem of weight loss and the long-range one of maintaining the loss:

By following the exercise and nutrition plans you can lose whatever number of pounds and inches are necessary.

You can maintain your correct weight permanently, without fighting to do so, and accomplish many other physical objectives if the Yoga exercises and principles of nutrition become a comfortable, meaningful part of your daily life.

Because of the *type* of movements that are involved, you will find Hatha Yoga the least intrusive method of exercising. The system feels completely natural because it conforms to the natural way in

12

which the body moves. Strain and fatigue are absent; therefore, it quickly and easily becomes a part of one's daily routine and is looked forward to as an activity that imparts strength, vitality, beauty and an elevation of spirit.

The life-force *(prana)* derived from the application of the Hatha Yoga techniques is of great magnitude and will provide the student with, among other things, the sustained incentive necessary to give the Yoga menus a fair trial. Once the effectiveness of these menus has been experienced—with regard to both the weight problem and general health—the student will certainly wish to consider Yoga Nutrition as a permanent approach to diet. Thus, another major basic change in the living pattern will have been established.

The results of these new patterns are usually so impressive that the student—now firmly on the way to realizing his physical goals—seeks to determine what other aspects of Yoga can be meaningful.

In this manner, many, many overweight people who have begun the practice of Yoga simply in the hope of losing pounds and inches have gradually found themselves involved in a totally new life, a life calculated not to conflict with one's basic beliefs but to impart expanded meaning to them; not to detract from the joy of living but to be highly additive. The truth of these statements will become self-evident as the student proceeds.

CHAPTER 2
WHAT MAKES IT WORK:
EXERCISE, NUTRITION AND
ENCOURAGEMENT

Exercise: The Hatha Yoga system is concerned not with the *amount* of movement, but with the *type* of movement. In utilizing slow motion, sustained "holds" and few repetitions, the Yoga exercises differ radically from those which constitute the familiar systems of calisthenics. With regard to the weight problem it is, therefore, not our objective to perspire away pounds and inches with many repetitions of quick movements; this is, at best, a partial, temporary and uncomfortable solution. There are often many physical as well as psychological factors involved in an overweight condition and the effectiveness of Yoga lies in its ability to exercise, methodically and thoroughly, *all* systems of the body. In addition to specific movements for reducing, redistributing and firming, you will perform breathing exercises for the respiratory system, apply quieting techniques to the nervous system and, with ingenious postures, stimulate the glands of the endocrine system.

Thus, while the Yoga exercises in this book are specially arranged so that they become practical for the overweight person, *obesity is not isolated as a particular condition to be dealt with, but is regarded as one of many problems that will respond to total exercising of the total organism.* When all is said and done, this "total" approach will prove to be the one which is most intelligent and most effective.

Nutrition: The Yoga Menus are to be used in conjunction with the exercise plan. All necessary information is given in Section Four.

14

Encouragement: The overweight person must be able to maintain his resolve for whatever period of time is necessary to achieve his objectives. "Will power" and "discipline" are words frequently used in connection with weight-loss plans. But these terms are inappropriate in our Yoga program, because the images evoked relate to a "split," a battle between a "good self" who is strong and must ride herd over a "bad self" who is weak. Such a "split" creates endless conflict and is responsible for the failure of many "self-improvement" ventures. In the practice of Yoga we find that we are not dealing with "good" and "bad," or "strong" and "weak" selves, but that we are of a single purpose and a single mind.

Your strongest source of encouragement in this plan will be, of course, the actual loss of weight. But there can be times when, for a multitude of reasons, your resolve may weaken and you begin to think about deviating from the program. This is a point at which other aspects of Yoga can be of great aid. For example, if the student has become familiar with the concepts of Hatha Yoga, the perfect functioning of his physical organism assumes the greatest possible importance. He is aware that more than health and appearance are at stake; an overweight condition inhibits the development of great potential forces with which Hatha Yoga deals. With this knowledge, the desire to regulate weight, as well as eliminate other negative physical conditions, is greatly intensified and this intensity is sustained.

Another aspect of Yoga, the practice of Meditation, wherein a profound self-introspection is undertaken, also serves to strengthen one's dedication. But in the event that you are not acquainted with these other aspects of Yoga, you can practice three excellent techniques that will be extremely helpful in maintaining your resolve at a high level and in quickly restoring your strength of purpose should it weaken. Although these three techniques will be performed as a part of your regular practice plan, each may be used *whenever necessary* for the purposes outlined below.

Recharging (both physical and psychic): When your energy is low you can become vulnerable to backsliding. If you experience such a let-down in vitality, it is possible to recharge the organism with the *Direction of Life-Force* technique, instructed on page 91.

Stabilizing the emotions: The overweight person's sudden need to eat is obviously not a real demand of the physical organism; his body is already bearing a taxing burden in the form of excess weight and hardly requires additional nourishment. It is most often an *emotional* need that sends the fatty scurrying to the refrigerator, hot-dog stand, candy shop, etc. We need not, at this point, be concerned with the cause of these emotional uprisings; we simply know that they create an imbalance in the organism. If equanimity can be quickly restored whenever necessary, those emotional conditions which, among other negative activities, result in compulsive eating will gradually subside and eventually no longer arise. There is genuine satisfaction and great subtle nourishment to be derived from certain breathing exercises.

Alternate Nostril Breathing, page 128 provides such nourishment and, in the course of satisfying emotional appetites, restores strength and equilibrium. If possible, this breathing technique should be done at the first sign of imaginary hungers.

Deep Relaxation: This exercise in quietude described on page 174, will help eliminate tensions from the body and negative thoughts from the mind. It puts us in direct communication with our life principle, contact with which is frequently lost amidst the frenzy of daily activities; we become more aware of our true natures, of our reflections of Spirit. Experiencing, through Deep Relaxation, a profound sense of peace that is carried over more and more into daily life, we are able to rise above many situations that might otherwise drain our life-force and cloud our objectives. Do not hesitate to use this or the other two techniques in meeting any physical, emotional or mental disturbance that may arise.

SECTION TWO

THE
OPTIONAL
FASTING PLANS

CHAPTER 1

YOU CAN LOSE UP TO 10% OF YOUR TOTAL WEIGHT DURING THE FIRST WEEK OF THE PROGRAM!

Depending upon your present weight, it is possible for you to lose up to 20 pounds in the first seven days of our program. This rapid weight loss is accomplished by following the exercise plan exactly as it is described and by utilizing the Yoga technique of *fasting*.

Fasting—partial or total abstinence from food—is a science that has been applied by Yogis for countless centuries to combat certain abnormal physical conditions. Obesity is one such condition; it is considered an illness, a disease. The cure is to eliminate the causes: too few of the proper activities and too many of the incorrect foods. The *total* exercising routines of Yoga will provide us with the "proper activities." Yoga Nutrition teaches us which foods offer the most real nourishment while simultaneously helping us to permanently regulate our weight.

Your appreciation of the genuine value of the Yoga Nutrition principles and your desire to incorporate them into your daily life can be greatly increased if a period of fasting is undertaken. This is because of the remarkable transformation that occurs in the body when it is given a short respite from food; the taste buds are purified and the entire organism regains its sensitivity to important sources of life-force that have been obscured by years of incorrect eating and living habits. Let us briefly examine the theory of fasting and learn how it can apply specifically to weight regulation.

Fasting is not starving. Fasting is voluntary abstinence from food, usually undertaken for a specific purpose. From the physical standpoint the Yogi fasts as part of a program of *regeneration:* cleansing and re-building. It is the theory of the Yogis (as well as numerous groups of health-minded people throughout the world) that when the digestive organs are permitted to rest, by virtue of the fast, a cleansing process is initiated. This process will continue as long as the fast is in effect. It is when this process has been completed (the completion being indicated by certain symptoms) that the fast is terminated. At this point unless food is again introduced into the organism, it will begin to feed upon itself; this marks the end of fasting and the beginning of starvation.

You may be surprised to learn that a long period of time can elapse from the beginning of the fast to that point when starvation begins. If psychologically prepared so that a false fear of starvation does not become a serious disturbance, most people can go for many weeks without food; two to three months is not unusual when a prolonged fast is undertaken. This is possible because the amount of food substances present in the organism at any given time is considerable. There are thousands of people throughout the United States and Europe who each year undertake a period of fasting for regenerative purposes.

A lengthy fast, however, is impractical for most working men and women because of long periods of rest and medical supervision that are advisable. But for overweight people a *short* fast is practical and highly beneficial. If you can indeed view your obesity not as an inconvenience in purchasing clothes or as a social handicap, but rather as a very real illness in which your entire organism suffers a continual, excessive, life-shortening stress and strain, the concept of fasting, of resting your digestive organs, will assume tremendous value. Yogis tell us that it is a form of insanity to continue to feed an already-bloated body; therefore, unless advised otherwise by your physician, you can attempt a seven-day partial or total fast beginning immediately. Following are three fasting plans from which you may choose:

20

CHAPTER 2

THE PARTIAL FAST

This is the mildest and most gradual of the fasting plans, but it will, nonetheless, result in a significant weight loss when undertaken in conjunction with the exercises. This plan is for people who are uncertain as to the effects of complete abstention from solid food and want to proceed cautiously.

The plan calls for total fasting on the first day (any person who is not seriously debilitated can fast for one full day with a minimum of discomfort), followed by six days of liquid lunches, and dinners consisting of light solid foods. Breakfasts are eliminated. Not eating before noon is an important feature of this plan. The Yogis believe that the morning is a time for resting the digestive organs. The elimination of breakfast allows several hours for the body to continue the cleansing process initiated during the previous night's sleep and greatly aids in weight reduction.

After several days you will experience no discomfort in going without breakfast, and following this first week, when you move into the "Transition Menus," you may find that you have lost all desire for breakfast and wish to eliminate it permanently. "No breakfast" means exactly that. It does not mean "just orange juice" or "just a cup of coffee." With the exception of water, if thirsty, you consume no food until the noon hour.

The liquid lunches that are indicated will provide sufficient nourishment to complete your afternoon's work. These drinks must be consumed *very slowly;* you should take 10 to 15 minutes to sip the contents of the glass. There is to be no eating, no snacks, between lunch and dinner. You drink spring water if thirsty.

Following the light dinners indicated there is no further eating (absolutely no bedtime snacks) until lunch the next day.

On the eighth day you begin the "Transition Menus" and follow them for three weeks. Then you move to the "Maintenance Menus" for completing and permanently maintaining your weight loss.

CHAPTER 3

PARTIAL FAST MENUS

The drinks and meals below are taken from the Transition and Maintenance Menus. Substitutions can be made from these menus if desired. If dinner substitutions are made, it is advisable not to include flesh foods. Be sure to read the information on menus in Section 4 before beginning the fast.

Breakfasts are eliminated. You drink spring water only if thirsty.

	LUNCH	DINNER	EXERCISE PLAN
1st Day	Fast	Fast	1A
2nd Day	Pineapple-Carrot Drink 1/2 cup pineapple juice 1/2 cup carrot juice 1 tsp. lemon 1 tsp. shredded coconut 1 tsp. brewers yeast Blend	Salad Napa cabbage, watercress, Bermuda onion. Dressing: lemon juice and olive oil. Casserole Mushrooms and brown rice. Fresh papaya	2A
3rd Day	Coconut-Banana Drink 1 banana 1/2 cup coconut juice 1 tbsp. wheat germ 2 dates (pitted) Blend	Salad Sliced tomatoes with basil. Cheese souffle (made with natural cheddar) Fruit compote (made with fresh fruits in season)	3A

4th Day	**Beet-Yogurt Drink**
	    2 beets
	    1 cup tomato
	    juice
	    1 tbsp. yogurt
	    1 tsp. parsley
	    Blend
		Salad
		    Romaine lettuce
		with parmesan cheese
		dressing.
		
		Whole wheat noodles
		with vegetarian tomato
		sauce.
		
		Honeydew melon
			1A

5th Day	**Date Milk**
	    1 cup non-fat milk
	    3 pitted, chopped
	    dates
	    1 tbsp. shredded
	    coconut
	    1 tsp. wheat germ
	    1 tsp. safflower oil
	
	    Blend
		Salad
		    Bell pepper; sliced,
		raw
		
		Approximately 3/4
		inch slice of baked egg-
		plant with ricotta cheese
		and tomato sauce
		
		Fruit gelatin made
		with fresh orange juice
			2A

6th Day	**Apple Drink**
	    1 cup pure apple
	    juice
	    1 tbsp. yogurt
	    1 tsp. brewers' yeast
	
	    Blend
		Bowl of lentil soup
		    (meatless)
		
		1/2 eggplant stuffed
		with sauteed onions
		and tomatoes and
		baked.
		
		Sherbet
		    Blend watermelon
		(or any soft, juicy
		fresh fruit in season)
		with sprig of mint.
		Freeze.
			3A

7th Day	**Energy Drink**
	    1/2 cup prune or
	    fig juice
	    1/2 cup apple juice
	    1 tsp. nut butter
	    1 tsp. yogurt
	    1 tsp. sesame or
	    safflower oil
	
	    Blend
		Pure tomato soup
		    Steam 3 tomatoes;
		blend in blender; add
		vegetable salt to taste.
		
		    Zucchini, grated and
		baked. Dot with mar-
		garine and sprinkle with
		parmesan cheese.
		
		Chunks of pineapple
		with yogurt
			Rest

8th Day—Continue the program with the Transition Menus for the next three weeks. Then move to the Maintenance Menus.

If you are away from home at lunch, it will be necessary to prepare the lunch drinks at home and take them with you in a container or thermos. At lunchtime shake the container vigorously for approximately one minute. Then drink *very slowly*.

CHAPTER 4

THE LIQUID FAST:
WHAT IS IT?

This fast is for people who desire a rapid weight loss but feel they cannot be without some food substances for a seven-day period.

The plan indicates one day of complete fasting followed by six days of the elimination of breakfast, a fruit or vegetable juice at lunch, a fruit or vegetable juice in the mid-afternoon, and a heavier blender drink for dinner. *All drinks are to be consumed very slowly.*

When this liquid fast is undertaken in conjunction with the exercise plan, a loss of approximately 7% of your total weight should result during the week.

If you complete this liquid fast, *you can bypass the Transition Menus and beginning the eighth day, move directly into the Maintenance Menus.* Follow these Maintenance Menus and the exercise plan faithfully and you should be able to attain your weight-loss objectives within the following 30 to 60 days.

For most people the Liquid Fast, rather than becoming more difficult, actually becomes easier as the days pass. If, however, at some point you feel you cannot continue the Liquid Fast, revert to the Partial Fast for the remainder of the week.

CHAPTER 5

LIQUID FAST MENUS

The drinks below are taken from the Transition and Maintenance Menus. Substitutions can be made from these menus if desired. Be sure to read the information on Menus in Section 4 before beginning the fast.

Breakfasts are eliminated. You drink spring water only if thirsty.

	LUNCH MID-AFTERNOON	DINNER	EXERCISE PLAN
1st Day	Fast	Fast	1A
2nd Day	Each noon and mid-afternoon drink 6-8 ozs. of any one of the following juices: Freshly squeezed orange or grapefruit; pure (unsweetened) grape, prune, fig or apple; Any single or combination of freshly squeezed vegetable juices.	Pineapple-Carrot Drink 1/2 cup pineapple juice 1/2 cup carrot juice 1 tsp. lemon 1 tsp. shredded coconut 1 tsp. brewers yeast Blend	2A
3rd Day	Same as Second Day	Coconut-Banana Drink 1 banana 1/2 cup coconut juice 1 tbsp. wheat germ 2 dates (pitted) Blend	3A

4th Day	Same	Beet-Yogurt Drink 2 beets 1 cup tomato juice 1 tbsp. yogurt 1 tsp. parsley Blend	1A
5th Day	Same	Date Milk 1 cup non-fat milk 3 pitted, chopped dates 1 tbsp. shredded coconut 1 tsp. wheat germ 1 tsp. safflower oil Blend	2A
6th Day	Same	Apple Drink 1 cup pure apple juice 1 tbsp. yogurt 1 tsp. brewers yeast Blend	3A
7th Day	Same	Energy Drink 1/2 cup prune or fig juice 1/2 cup apple juice 1 tsp. nut butter 1 tsp. yogurt 1 tsp. sesame or safflower oil Blend	REST

8th Day—Continue the program with the Maintenance Menus on a permanent basis.

If you do not have access to freshly squeezed or pure fruit and vegetable juices at lunchtime or in the mid-afternoon, it will be necessary to take these drinks with you in a container. Before drinking, shake the container well; *drink very slowly.*

CHAPTER 6
THE TOTAL FAST

An immediate and dramatic weight loss results from the Total Fast. When it is undertaken in conjunction with the exercise plan, up to 10% of your total weight will be lost in seven days!

The Total Fast means, in this program, complete abstinence from food for one week; for example, if the fast begins on Sunday night with the elimination of dinner, it is broken with dinner the following Sunday night. You drink spring water only when thirsty.

Total Fasting is for those overweight people who have an urgent need to take off pounds and inches as quickly as possible, who are strongly attracted to the "idea" and "feeling" of a total fast and who have confidence in their ability to sustain the fast if certain minor discomforts are experienced. If these are not present in the individual, it is best that he proceed with one of the other two milder forms of fasting.

The Total Fast is *not to exceed one week*. It is broken on the eighth day by using the Maintenance Menus and continuing with these menus on a permanent basis.

As with the Liquid Fast, the Total Fast, for most people, becomes easier as the days of the week pass. The first 48 hours are usually the most difficult. After these first two days you will probably find that the subsequent five days are relatively easy. If, however, at some point in this Total Fast you feel you cannot continue, revert to the Liquid Fast or, if necessary, the Partial Fast for the remainder of the week.

Here is the exercise plan that you follow during the fasting week: *1st Day*—1A; *2nd Day*—2A; *3rd Day*—3A; *4th Day*—1A; *5th Day*—2A; *6th Day*—3A; *7th Day*— Rest.

CHAPTER 7

QUESTIONS & ANSWERS
ON THE THREE FASTING PLANS

Here are the answers to the four most frequently asked questions by people contemplating a fast:

Q. If I fast, won't I be terribly hungry all the time?

A. No. Actually no overweight person is ever really hungry. Despite the excessive amounts of food he craves and is able to consume, he is already so overfed that it is not hunger which he experiences. *Real* hunger occurs, somewhat like thirst, in the mouth and throat, not the stomach. When you abstain from, or significantly reduce your intake of food, the bloated stomach begins to shrink, giving rise to the false "hunger pangs." This emptiness, which is actually greeted with great relief by the body, is interpreted by the mind as a form of deprivation; it distorts the emptiness and enlarges it, out of all proportion, into a serious discomfort, often as a major threat to life itself.

If, however, during the first day or two of a fast, especially the Total Fast, you can become sensitive to the true condition of your body, if you can "tune in" to what it is saying, you will perceive that it is not really suffering and is certainly not threatened. It is the *mind* that is hungry! After the first few days of a fast the hunger pangs usually diminish to the point where they are no longer bothersome. The Yoga exercise routines, which include the Complete Breath and relaxation techniques, help to quiet the mind and relieve it of its hunger anxieties. This is why, for most students, fasting has become easier as the week passes. I have known people who, in their thirtieth day of total fasting have not experienced any hunger whatsoever since their first week! (Remember that prolonged fasting is not a part of this program.)

Q. If I don't eat, won't I be too weak to do my work?

A. Ideally, the time to fast is when you can rest as frequently as you desire, when pressures and obligations are at a minimum. But in my view, overweight people cannot afford to wait for "ideal" conditions. They need to lose weight *now*. Therefore, the fasts of about 90% of my overweight students are undertaken in the context of their usual activities—jobs, housework, social obligations, etc. Yes, there will be periods of weakness, the intensity of which will depend on which of the fasts you follow. But these periods will be brief; they prevent very few persons from carrying on with their work. The weakness is not caused directly by a lack of food. It is due to the cleansing process that is initiated when the fast begins. At certain intervals the body works exceptionally hard at this cleansing process and at reducing its excess weight. It is at these times that an uncomfortable weakness can occur. Usually these periods pass quickly. Since no two people react identically to the fast, there is no way of predicting with certainty how much or how little activity you will find comfortable. It is very seldom that work which is essential is interrupted by the fast. However, during the fasting week it is advisable to arrange for a minimum of activity when the day's work is completed.

If you undertake the Liquid or Total Fast, the hours may seem to pass quite slowly from the time you finish work until the next morning. Some students have found that staying busy with light activities that do not require much energy or talking is helpful. Others prefer complete rest. The rule is simply to do whatever you find more comfortable. It is interesting to note that while fasting, many students have lengthy periods wherein they feel more alert and have more energy than when they are eating! This may seem strange to one who has never fasted but it is, nonetheless, a fact which, in all probability you will experience.

Q. If I skip a meal, I get a headache and feel nauseated. What causes this?

A. The same cleansing process explained above. This first-day headache usually lasts several hours and then disappears. In most cases, once gone, the headache does not return. Nausea, if it should occur, usually passes within minutes. Suffer through these minor discomforts; they won't be so bad and, when compared with the results we can achieve, are of little consequence. Under no circumstances must you take any medication for these symptoms. (Let me reiterate that unless prescribed by your physician, absolutely no drugs or patent medicines of any kind are to be used in this program. No laxatives are to be taken; all necessary elimination will occur naturally.)

In addition to periods of weakness, an initial headache, and possibly a brief nausea, other minor discomforts can occur in the Liquid or Total Fast. For example, on certain nights of the fast you may have a restless sleep. Also, you may find yourself somewhat irritable from time to time during the week. If you understand that these also must be attributed to the cleansing process, in which poisons that have been stored in the organism are now being passed into blood for elimination, their discomforts can be borne more easily. Indeed, such symptoms are actually to be welcomed since, for us, they are positive indications of cleansing and reducing. Almost all of these discomforts will respond well to several Complete Breaths and/or practice of the relaxation exercises that are listed under "Controlling the Mind and Emotions." If you find yourself feeling physically uncomfortable or emotionally "on edge," try to get away from your activities for a few minutes; do the complete breathing and, if your surroundings permit, one of the relaxation exercises.

During your lunch hour and other "breaks," go off by yourself, do some complete breathing and rest quietly for a few minutes. The less talking you do during the fast, the more energy you'll have. If you work at home, you can follow the above suggestions several times during the day.

If you smoke during the fast you will artificially increase all of the possible discomforts: hunger pangs, irritability, headaches, insomnia, and nausea. To smoke in general is to court disaster; smoking during a fast is immediately self-defeating.

Q. I have to do the cooking for my family. Won't it be difficult for me to fast?

A. Other than the foods and liquids that are being consumed according to the fasting plan, it is certainly ideal that you have as little contact as possible with the sight and odor of food during the fasting week. But if this is not possible, if you cannot avoid your cooking chores (and this is the case with most of our students who are housewives), then adhering to any one of the three fasting plans will certainly require an extra effort on your part. And if you undertake the Partial Fast, you may have to prepare one type of meal for the family and another for yourself.

But you must realize that your obesity is a disease that affects your life negatively on every level. Surely only one week of extra effort and resolve is a small price to pay for what can be accomplished. Simply decide *now* to do it. Mention to your family that you are on a special one-week "diet" and stick with your resolution. (Incidentally, "diet" is an acceptable word; "fasting" is an eyebrow-raiser.) Attempt to serve more simple meals to your family that require a minimum of preparation and tasting on your part during that week. With determination and the slightest bit of ingenuity, you will be able to solve any problem that arises.

CHAPTER 8

OTHER HELPFUL HINTS WHILE FASTING

• When breaking the one-week fast, especially the Liquid or Total Fast, you must be very much on your guard *not to overeat*. Following the Transition or Maintenance Menus exactly as indicated will prevent this from happening.

You must not be alarmed when you regain several pounds in the first days of the week following the Liquid or Total Fast. This is natural and is taken into account in the program. The weight gain will level off in a few days and then the losing process will be resumed. Remember: you must adhere to the Transition or Maintenance Menus (whichever is indicated) when the fast is broken to insure a continued loss of weight even though several pounds are regained in the first few days following the fast. One of the major objectives of the fast is to make the permanent adoption of these menus easy, once the fast is broken.

• Absolutely no appetite depressants of any kind are to be used. We want to aid, not inhibit, nature in regulating our weight. Pills, powders, wafers and liquids that act to "kill" the appetite are in direct conflict with our objectives in this program.

• The exercises are done daily, regardless of whether or not you are fasting. If you have the time, additional benefits are frequently derived from practicing the daily exercise plan *twice* during the day. The "A" routines that you will be doing during the fasting week are so mild that you should experience no difficulty in performing them. Often, a student who is fasting and feels somewhat weak before beginning the exercises regains his energy and strengthens his determination simply by performing the exercise plan of the day. If you are away from home during the day, the best time to practice is in the early evening.

• We want to consume as little fluid as possible, in addition to that which is indicated in the fasting menus. For this reason we drink water only when we are really thirsty. We prefer small amounts of spring water (that is, water without the chemical additives that are present in most tap water). You can purchase this water in large or small bottles from water companies or in many markets. Most offices have bottled spring water. Sip your water slowly. In all probability you will very seldom be thirsty during the Partial or Liquid Fast. However, after the first day or two of the Total Fast, you may need water every two to three hours. Some fasting authorities advise the drinking of a glass of water at regular intervals. This is not the case in our program. We drink small amounts of water, very slowly, only when we experience a real thirst in the mouth and throat (not an emptiness in the stomach).

• It is imperative that you speak as little as possible to friends, relatives and co-workers regarding your fast. Much of the value of the fast can be dissipated if you engage in discussions about it. If people notice that you are eating lightly or not eating at all, you must dismiss the subject with as few words as possible. Any polite excuse that will not encourage further questioning will do. Actually the entire Yoga weight-loss program is best left without discussion. When you achieve your final objectives, you can speak about what you have been doing. From a great deal of experience I caution you against dissipating your energy through discussion while in the crucial stages of this program.

• In this text we are emphasizing the value of fasting for weight reduction. However, because of the cleansing process that occurs during the fast, students often find that certain minor aches and pains, respiratory difficulties and complexion problems are among the physical conditions that respond positively to the week's fast.

• After having experienced the benefits of the one-week fast, many thousands of our students continue to fast *one* day *each week*. They generally choose that day on which they have the least activities or social obligations. (It is desirable to choose the same day each week if possible so that a fasting "rhythm" is developed.) This regular one-day fast not only helps to insure maintenance of the weight loss but becomes a factor in the process of continual *regeneration* which is one of the major objectives of the entire Yoga practice.

•A few words regarding the spiritual aspect of fasting are in order here. You are probably aware that in the scriptures of most major religions throughout the world, there are allusions to "fasting." I have found that many people think of fasting, in its spiritual context, as a form of denial, discipline, penance or punishment. This is not the case, especially from the Yogic viewpoint. During the fast there is most often a sensation of elation and spirituality that is difficult to explain and really must be experienced to be understood. But as one ceases to eat, the physical aspect of his existence temporarily becomes less of a reality and he is increasingly aware of his spiritual nature. Such awareness can be described as "exhilarating," "inspiring," "joyous." All of the great saints and religious leaders throughout history have utilized the fast to gain inspiration and spiritual insight. The Yogi believes that a period of fasting should always precede or be undertaken in conjunction with deep meditation. We mention these things here so that you will understand there is more involved in fasting than weight loss or physical regeneration.

• It is not essential to fast in this weight-loss program to achieve your objectives. Your reduction of pounds and inches will be sure, steady and permanent if you follow the exercise plan in conjunction with menus, as advised. The fasting plans are offered as an *adjunct* to the program whereby the weight loss can be accelerated and through which the Yoga Nutrition principles and menus become easy to adopt because of the transformation that occurs in the body during the fast. Accordingly, if you are not attracted by the idea of fasting or if you feel it presents too many difficulties, simply proceed with the exercise plan and the Transition Menus *now*.

• Before undertaking any part of this program, including the fasting plans, make certain to consult your physician if:
  • you are currently under his care;
  • you are taking prescribed drugs;
  • you are more than 75 pounds overweight;
  • you have a history of serious illness.

It is always advisable to receive the permission of your physician before beginning any weight-loss program.

THE
EXERCISE
ROUTINES

THE THREE EXERCISE ROUTINES

The Yoga exercises for our weight-loss program are grouped into three Routines: 1, 2 and 3. Each Routine serves for one day's practice and covers four essential aspects of weight loss.

The first group of each day's exercise Routine is for reducing—losing pounds and trimming inches. These reducing exercises are performed in *continuous slow motion*.

With the second group of each day's exercise Routine, you will firm and restore excellent muscle tone. These are also performed in slow motion but we will also *hold the extreme positions motionless*. This "holding" technique intensifies the firming and strengthening qualities of the exercises.

The third group of each day's Routine is composed of movements that will stimulate organs and glands.

The fourth group contains techniques for strengthening your resolve, for helping to gain control of your mind and emotions, so that you can maintain your dedication to a successful conclusion of the program.

Here is a complete list of the exercises as you will perform them in the three Routines:

	ROUTINE 1	ROUTINE 2	ROUTINE 3
Reducing	Complete Breath Side Bend Cobra Bow Lie Down; Sit Up	Complete Breath Triangle Twist Leg Over Chin Exercise	Complete Breath Rishi's Posture Dancer's Posture Roll Twist Seated Side Bend
Firming	Leg Clasp Side Raise	Back Stretch Shoulder Raise Locust	Lion Alternate Leg Pull Back Push-Up
Stimulating organs and glands	Abdominal Exercises	Head Stand	Shoulder Stand
Controlling mind and emotions	Direction of the Life-Force	Alternate Nostril Breathing	Deep Relaxation

Most of the above Yoga exercises have elementary, intermediate and advanced positions; this is the key to the entire plan. You will progress from one group of positions to the next according to your weight loss. Let us designate your present weight as stage "A." When you have lost approximately half of the weight you want to lose you will be in stage "B." When you are approximately 5 to 10 pounds away from the total number of pounds you want to lose, you will be in stage "C." For example, if your present weight is 200 pounds, and you need to reduce to 160 pounds (a reduction of 40 pounds), then: "A" = 200 pounds; "B" = 185-180 pounds; "C" = 165-160 pounds.

In the following pages you will note that the exercises designated as "A" depict the elementary movements. You will use these in the beginning stage of the program when you are at your heaviest. By carefully following the instructions of "A" you will be able to undertake effective exercising regardless of how heavy you are. There will be a minimum of exertion. *You must practice only the movements of "A" in each exercise until you have reached your intermediate stage. Do not move prematurely to the exercises of "B."*

The "B" positions depict the intermediate movements of the exercises and are for use when you have lost approximately half of your intended weight. You may reach this stage in as brief a period as one to two weeks. At this intermediate point you will eliminate the "A" movements since the loss of pounds and inches will enable you to move into the "B" positions. During this intermediate stage of the program, you practice only the "B" movements. Do not attempt the movements of "C."

"C" depicts the advanced movements and is for use when you are approximately 5 to 10 pounds from your final goal. At this point you will eliminate the "B" movements since your additional loss of pounds and inches now allows you to perform the "C" positions.

These advanced movements will not only help you to achieve your final weight objective, but will serve as a lifetime plan of maintenance. In other words, having once normalized your weight and figure, you continue with the "C" movements for permanent weight regulation and control.

HOW YOGA WEIGHT LOSS
WORKED FOR REAL PEOPLE

The photographs that follow show several of our subjects in the three stages of various exercises.

This subject began the program at 220 pounds. He lost 55 pounds and 37 1/4 inches in slightly more than three months. Eighteen pounds were lost in the first week! He now weighs 165.

BACK STRETCH

Subject, performing the "A" positions exactly as instructed, experiences a minimum of discomfort. In Yoga, it is the type of movement, not the amount of movement, that proves most effective.

Through patient and regular practice subject has lost 28 pounds and now performs "B" positions.

Advanced positions enable subject to complete and maintain loss of 55 pounds.

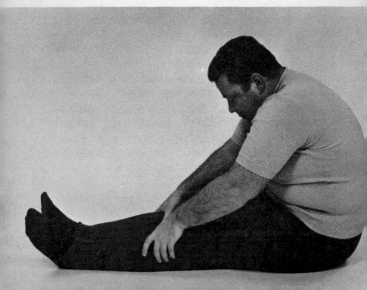

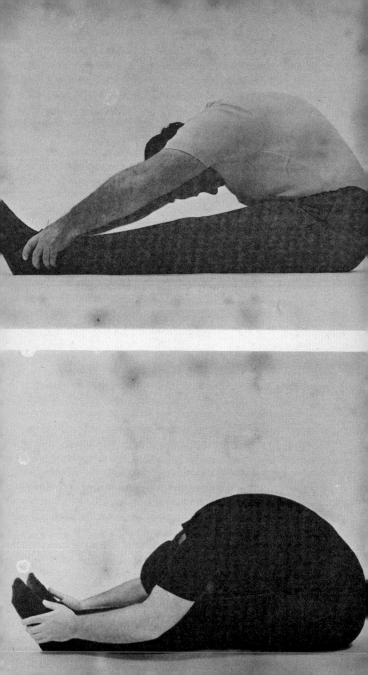

HEAD STAND

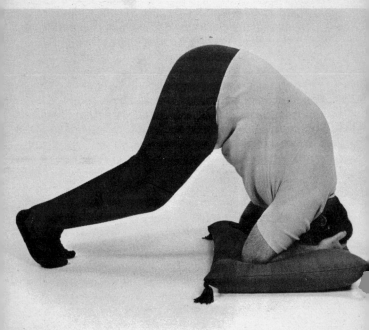

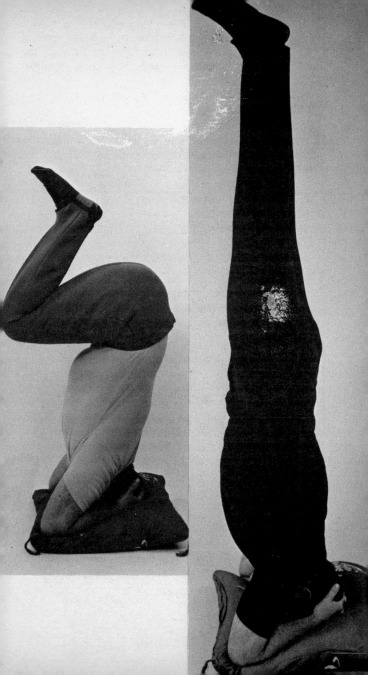

Women **subjects** illustrate how progressive loss of pounds and inches enables them to move through the three stages of the exercises—and show great improvement in their figures!

COMPLETE BREATH

Loss of weight in the legs permits this woman to achieve the Half-Lotus posture in stage "B" and the Full-Lotus in "C."

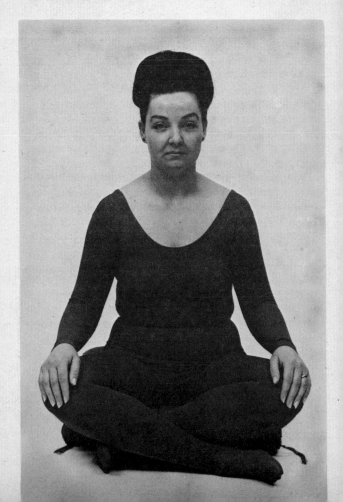

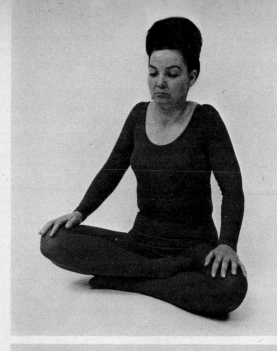

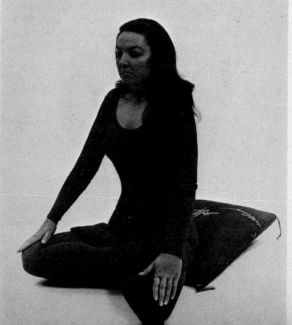

LEG CLASP

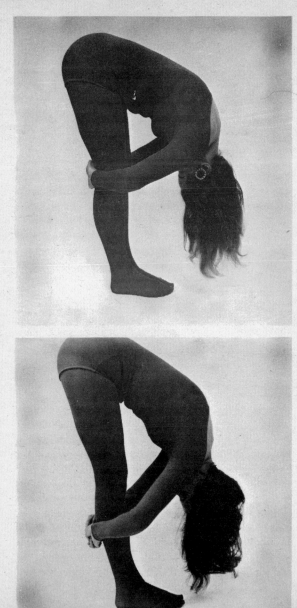

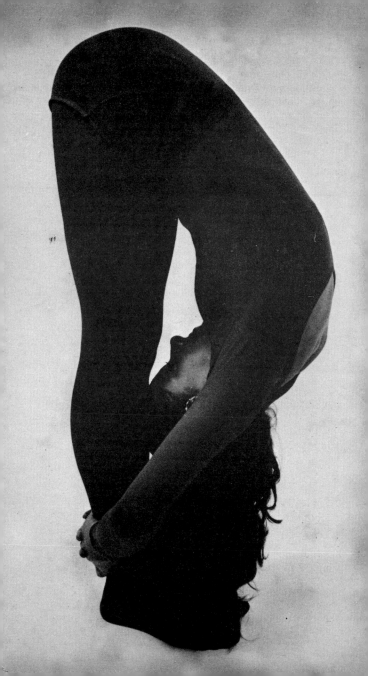

LEG OVER

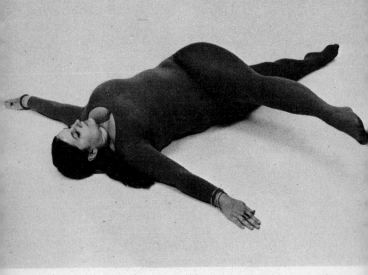

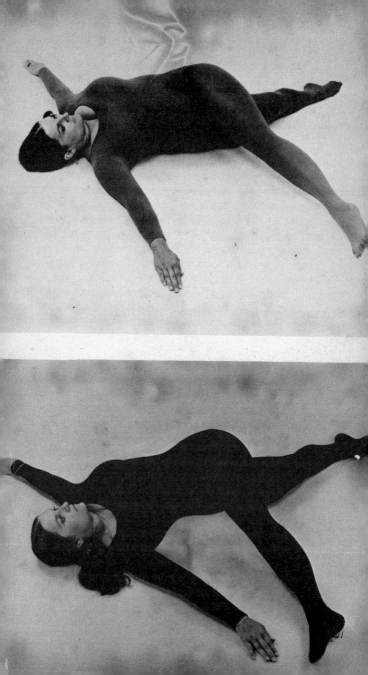

SHOULDER RAISE

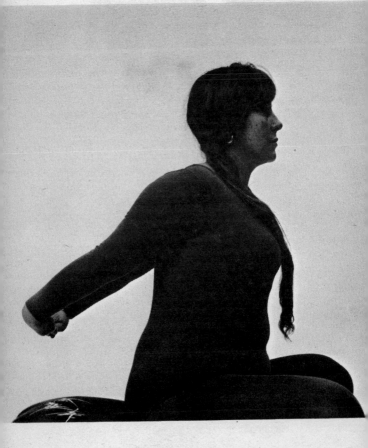

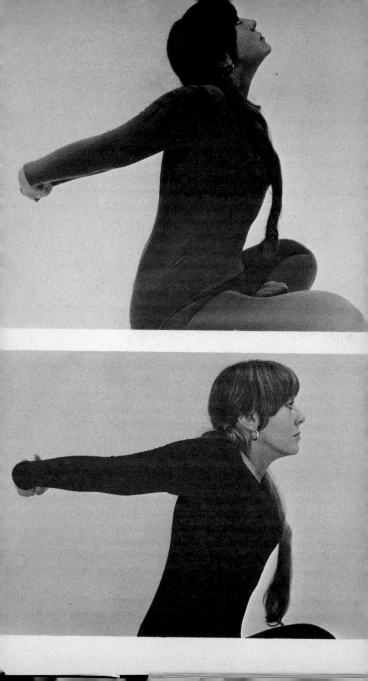

ADAPTING THE PROGRAM
TO YOUR PERSONAL NEEDS

If you need to lose:	Do the "A" exercises until you have lost approximately:	Then do the "B" exercises until you have lost approximately:
55-60 lbs.	20-30 lbs.	40-50 total lbs.
45-50 lbs.	18-25 lbs.	30-40 total lbs.
35-40 lbs.	15-20 lbs.	25-30 total lbs.
25-30 lbs.	12-15 lbs.	18-23 total lbs.
15-20 lbs.	7-10 lbs.	12-15 total lbs.
5-10 lbs.		* Attempt to begin the program with the "B" exercises until 5 lbs. are lost.

Then complete your weight loss and maintain the loss with the "C" exercises.

In the event that you are no more than 5-10 pounds overweight, you may bypass "A" and begin the program with the "B" positions. However, if strain or discomfort results from beginning with "B," revert to the "A" positions until they become comfortable. Then move into the "B" and "C" positions according to your ability.

The transition from "A" to "B" to "C" should occur smoothly in accordance with your loss of weight. However, due to certain features of body structure, previous lack of activity, age, etc., some of the positions called for in the exercises of "B" or "C" may require a longer period for accomplishment. If this is the case, simply revert to the easier position of "A" or "B" for those particular exercises. Your body will soon be ready for the more advanced movements.

Each of the three routines listed on page 39 serves for one day's practice. The routines are continually rotated. For example, if you began your exercising on a Monday, you would use Routine 1; then on Tuesday, Routine 2; Wednesday, Routine 3; Thursday, back to Routine 1; Friday, Routine 2, etc. *Each seventh day you do not exercise,* you allow your body to rest and "set." On the following day you begin again with Routine 1, etc. So that you always know the correct routine for any given day, you must keep a simple, accurate record of your practice on a separate sheet of paper:

YOUR OWN YOGA
EXERCISE CHART

Fill in the day of the week that you start the exercises and follow by listing consecutive days of the week.

DAY OF WEEK   **ROUTINE**
(Do "A," "B" or "C" exercises, according to your weight)

_____	Routine 1
_____	Routine 2
_____	Routine 3
_____	Routine 1
_____	Routine 2
_____	Routine 3
_____	Rest
_____	Routine 1
_____	Routine 2
_____	Routine 3
_____	Routine 1
_____	Routine 2
_____	Routine 3
_____	Rest

It is essential to perform your exercises each day as scheduled. If for some absolutely unavoidable reason you are forced to miss a day, take up at the point where you left off on the following day. Remember, however, if you want the best results, you must make every effort to follow your schedule on the six consecutive days.

Each routine will require 20-30 minutes and must be done in its entirety. Each exercise has its own particular importance and none can be neglected even though, initially, it may require extra effort to perform correctly.

You will derive the greatest benefits from your practice sessions by conforming with the following:

• Select a well-ventilated area where distractions are at a minimum. The Yoga movements require a flat surface and sufficient space to stretch your trunk and limbs in all directions without interference.

• Cover your practice surface with a large towel, mat or pad. This cover is put away after exercising and is used only for Yoga.

• Your exercise clothing should allow for complete freedom of movement. Remove watch, eyeglasses and whatever may restrict your movement. Keep watch or clock handy for timing certain exercises.

• You can practice before eating (stomach empty) but wait at least 90 minutes following meals. Anytime of day is satisfactory.

• If in doubt regarding the effect of the Yoga techniques consult your physician before undertaking this or any weight-loss program.

• The Yoga exercises are performed in a series of graceful, rhythmic slow-motion movements with a brief "holding" (that is, completely motionless) period for certain of the extreme positions. Poise and balance are maintained at all times and your attention is fixed unwaveringly on the movements being executed. Therefore, make every attempt to approach each practice session in a serene frame of mind, having temporarily put aside all thoughts and activities that might be distracting.

ROUTINE 1

COMPLETE BREATH

Obesity usually causes a person to breathe shallowly with only the upper part of the lungs being utilized. The Yogic Complete Breath that we are about to learn makes use of the lungs to their fullest capacity, and you will find that this can have a very direct and immediate effect on both your health and weight. Bringing a greater volume of air into your organism provides increased life-force (prana), and it is astonishing how this aids our weight-loss objective. Not only are there the noticeable physical effects, but you will experience a strengthening of the emotions and "resolve" that enables you to undertake the plan of this book with a very positive attitude.

It is important to learn and practice the Complete Breath exactly as directed; you will have many occasions throughout your lifetime to resort to its practice. During fasting periods the Complete Breath should be done frequently.

(A) 1. Sit on your mat in this simple cross-legged position. Your ankles are crossed and your feet brought in toward you as far as is comfortable.

Work your abdominal muscles to gain some control of them. First, attempt to distend the abdomen (that is, push it out even farther than it is now protruding), and then contract (pull in) as far as possible. Perform these push and pull movements until you achieve some definite motion in the abdomen.

Now begin a slow exhalation through your nose (all breathing is done through the nose); simultaneously contract your abdomen, as just practiced, until your lungs feel completely empty.

Begin a very slow, quiet inhalation and simultaneously distend your abdomen as just practiced (this pushing out of the abdomen allows the air to enter the lower area of your lungs—something that is extremely valuable in obesity).

59

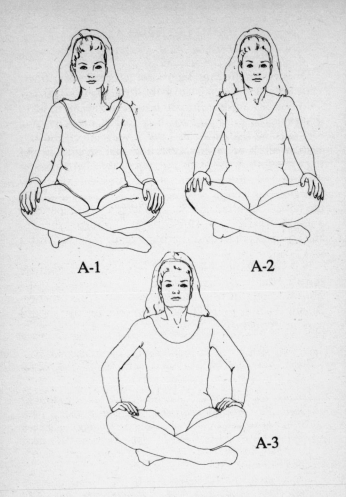

A-1   A-2

A-3

2. **Continue the slow, quiet, deep inhalation.** *Contract your abdomen slightly and simultaneously expand your chest.*

3. **Continue the slow, quiet, deep inhalation.** *Now slowly raise your shoulders as high as possible. This movement aids in allowing the air to enter the high area of the lungs.*

When your deep inhalation is completed, begin a slow, quiet, deep exhalation. Allow all muscles to relax during this exhalation. At the end of the exhalation contract the abdomen to help empty your lungs and then, without pause, begin the next slow, quiet, deep inhalation.

Perform 5 Complete Breaths in continuous motion.

All breathing is very slow and very quiet. Practice to make the movements **flow** into one another. Your eyes can be closed to help keep your full attention on the movements.

(B) 1. *There are no changes in the movements of the Complete Breath during your intermediate stages of weight loss. However, at this point you should be able to assume a more advanced seated posture—the Half-Lotus.*

*Your hands place your left foot as illustrated. The heel has been drawn in as far as possible and your left foot rests **against**, not under, your right thigh.*

2. *The completed Half-Lotus. Your right foot can be placed on top of the left thigh; or, if you prefer, in the cleft of the left leg. You can also attempt the Half-Lotus with your legs reversed to determine which is the more comfortable postion.*

The second movement of the Complete Breath is depicted in this illustration. Remember, you are performing all of the identical movements of the Complete Breath as previously learned in (A), but now you are seated in the Half-Lotus.

Perform 5 Complete Breaths.

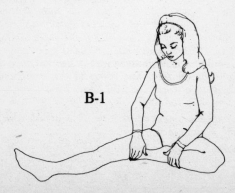

B-1

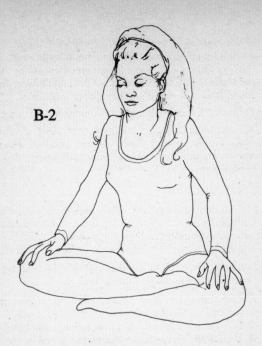

B-2

(C) 1. There are no changes in the movements of the Complete Breath during the final stages of weight loss. However, we can now presume that sufficient weight has been lost in the legs, thighs and abdomen to attempt the Full-Lotus.

Place your left foot as high as possible on your right thigh.

2. The completed Lotus. Place your right foot on top of the left thigh. Also attempt the Full-Lotus with your legs reversed to determine which is the more comfortable position. This is a difficult and advanced posture that can usually be accomplished with patient practice. If it is not possible at this time, revert to the Half-Lotus but continue to attempt the Full-Lotus from time to time. At some point you will be able to "slip" into it.

The final movement of the Complete Breath is depicted in this illustration.

Perform 5 Complete Breaths.

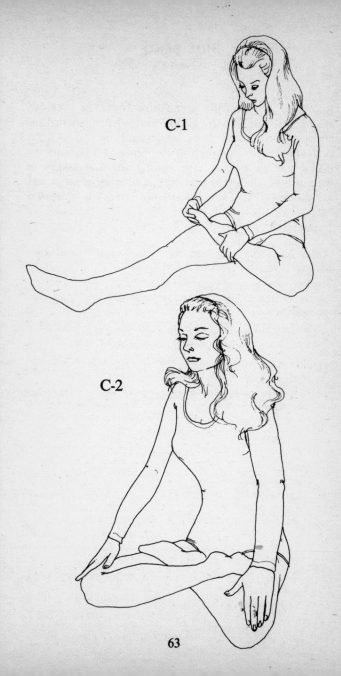

C-1

C-2

SIDE BEND
(To trim inches from the hips)

Stand up as gracefully as possible from the previous seated position. Each of our movements (including sitting down, lying down and standing up) will be performed with as much grace, poise and balance as possible. This is true even during the first stages of weight loss when you may feel at your most awkward and clumsy. If you will always move with the indicated "grace" you will find your body quickly beginning to resume its former shape and beauty!

(A) *1. Stand with your heels together. Gracefully raise arms overhead; palms face each other.*

Very slowly *bend your trunk and head a short distance to the left. Do not go farther than illustrated. Arms remain parallel.*

2. Without pause, straighten to the upright position and ***very slowly*** *bend an identical distance to the right.*

Perform 10 times in continuous slow motion. Slowly lower arms to the sides and relax for a few moments.

Remember, ***slow motion.*** *If you catch yourself hurrying, slow down.*

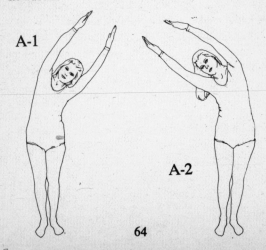

A-1

A-2

(B) 1. Very slowly bend an intermediate distance to the left. (Compare with A-1.) Do not go farther than illustrated. Arms remain parallel.

2. Without pause, slowly straighten to the upright position and very slowly bend an identical distance to the right.

Perform 10 times in continuous slow motion. Slowly lower arms to the sides and relax.

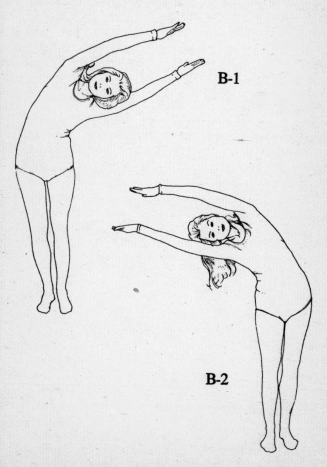

B-1

B-2

(C) 1. *Very slowly bend to the extreme left position. Arms must remain parallel.*

2. *Without pause, straighten to the upright position and very slowly bend to the extreme right position.*

Perform 10 times in continuous slow motion. Slowly lower arms to the sides and relax.

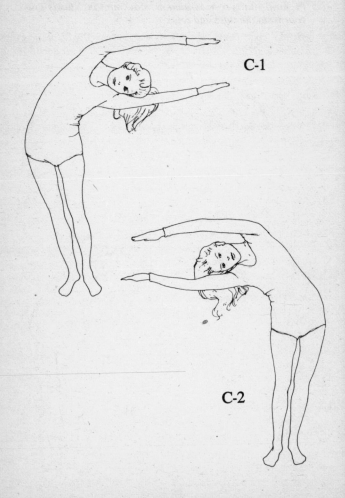

C-1

C-2

COBRA
(To trim inches from the trunk and buttocks)

Lie down as gracefully as possible from the previous standing position.

(A) 1. *Rest your forehead on your mat, arms at sides. Relax your body; do not hold any muscles tensed.*

Bring your arms up slowly and gracefully from your sides and place them beneath your shoulders as illustrated. Note the position of the hands: fingers are together and pointing at **right angles** *to the shoulders.*

2. **In very slow motion** *begin to raise your head and bend it backward.*

Push against the floor with your hands and begin to raise your trunk.

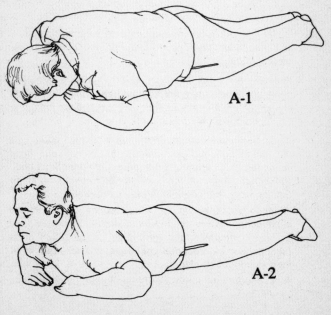

A-1

A-2

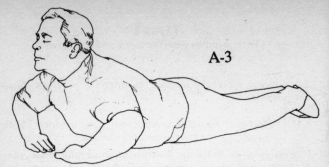

3. *In very slow motion* continue to raise your trunk to the position illustrated. Do not go farther. Note that your head bends backward and your spine is continually curved as you rise.

Without pause, in very slow motion, reverse the movements and lower your trunk until your forehead rests on the floor.

Without pause, repeat and perform 5 times in continuous slow motion. Upon completion rest your cheek on the mat and allow your body to go completely limp.

(B) 1. *Bend your head backward and raise your trunk slowly, as high as possible without the aid of your hands. (Arms remain at sides.)*

2. *When the trunk has been raised as high as possible, bring the arms up gracefully and smoothly and place the hands beneath the shoulders as we have done previously. Do not allow the trunk to lower.*

3. *In very slow motion continue to raise your trunk with the hands now pushing against the floor. Your head bends far backward and your spine is continually curved. Raise your trunk to the position illustrated. Do not go farther (note that your elbows are still bent).*

Without pause, in very slow motion, begin the reverse movements. When you have lowered approximately halfway, smoothly and gracefully bring your arms back to your sides so that your back muscles must work hard to support your trunk.

Now continue to lower slowly until your forehead rests on the floor.

Without pause, repeat and perform 5 times in continuous slow motion. Upon completion rest your cheek on the mat and allow your body to go completely limp.

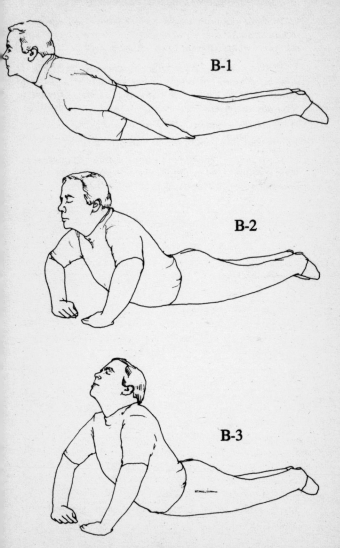

B-1

B-2

B-3

(C) Perform the identical movements of 1 and 2 under (B).

1. Now raise your trunk to the extreme position illustrated. Elbows are straight at this point.

2. Without pause, bend your right elbow (left elbow remains straight) and slowly twist your trunk as far to the left as possible. Attempt to see your left heel.

3. Without pause, slowly return to the position of Fig. 1; now bend your left elbow (right remains straight) and slowly twist as far to the right as possible. Attempt to see your right heel.

Without pause return to the position of Fig. 1.

Lower your forehead to the floor as practiced in (B).

Without pause, repeat and perform 3 times in continuous slow motion. Upon completion rest your cheek on the mat and allow your body to go completely limp.

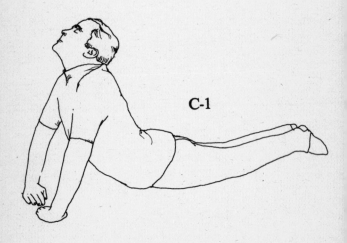

C-1

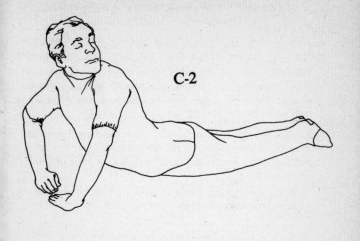

C-2

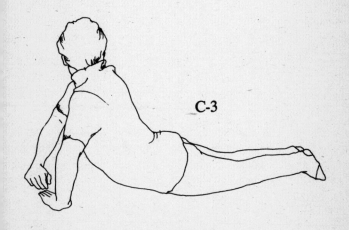

C-3

BOW
(To reduce the waist, back, thighs and buttocks)

(A) 1. *Rest your **chin** on the mat. Bend your knees, bring feet toward back. Reach behind you and attempt to hold your feet. Since in the initial stages of weight reduction it is often difficult to hold the feet directly, this illustration depicts how two towels (handkerchiefs, cloths, etc.) are utilized to aid the holding.*

2. *Slowly and cautiously raise your head and trunk a very moderate distance. Pull hard against your feet and perhaps your knees can also be raised an inch or two. Do not strain.*

Without pause very slowly lower knees, trunk and chin to floor; retain the hold on your feet. Without pause, repeat.

Perform 5 times in continuous slow motion. Upon completion release your feet and lower them to the floor. Rest your cheek on the mat and relax.

A-1

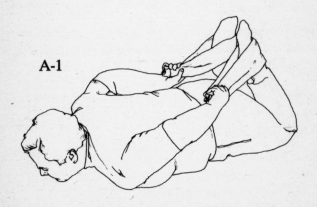

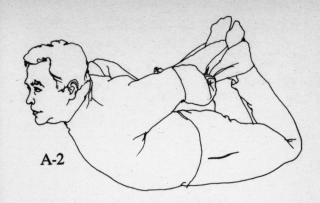

A-2

(B) 1. The feet are held firmly without the aid of the towels and the knees are now placed close together.

2. Pull hard against the feet and raise your head, trunk and knees a moderate distance. Do not go farther than illustrated. Attempt to keep the knees close together. These movements must be executed slowly and cautiously so that no strain is experienced.

Without pause very slowly lower knees, trunk and chin to floor; retain the hold on your feet. Without pause, repeat.

Perform 5 times in continuous slow motion. Upon completion release your feet and lower them to the floor (always move slowly and with grace). Rest your cheek on the mat and relax.

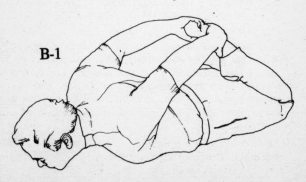

B-1

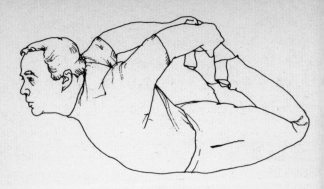

B-2

(C) 1. The trunk and knees are now slowly and cautiously raised to their limit. Your head is back and your knees are held as close together as possible.

*2. We now attempt to "rock" forward and backward on the abdomen in a hobby-horse movement. Therefore, hold your feet very firmly and rock **forward**, bringing your chin as close to the floor as possible.*

*3. Without pause rock **backward**, bringing your knees as close to the floor as possible.*

Perform these rocking movements 5 times in continuous slow motion, moving as smoothly (without jerking) as possible.

It is important to come out of the posture smoothly. When the rocking movements are completed, return to the extreme position of 1 and stop all motion for a moment. Then lower your knees to the floor first. Next, slowly lower your chin. Finally, release your feet and lower your legs slowly to the floor. Rest cheek on mat and relax.

Perform the entire routine of 1, 2, 3 three times. (This will make 15 rocking movements in all.)

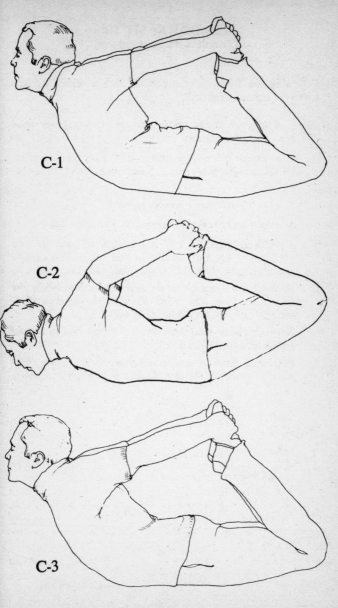

C-1

C-2

C-3

LIE DOWN; SIT UP
(To reduce the waist and legs)

Following the Bow, move gracefully into a seated posture with your legs outstretched.

(A) 1. Grip your thighs firmly and very slowly lower your back toward the floor.

2. Continue the slow lowering until your back rests on the floor. Without pause bring your knees in as illustrated.

3. Slowly straighten your legs upward.

4. Lower legs to the floor as slowly as possible.

5. Without pause, tense your abdominal muscles and use them as much as possible to help you into an upright seated position. Use your hands to aid you as necessary.

*Without pause take hold of your calves, just below the knees, and pull your trunk down to the position illustrated. Note that the elbows bend **outward**.*

Without pause straighten to the upright position and repeat the entire routine.

Perform 5 times in continuous slow motion. Upon completion return to the upright seated position and relax.

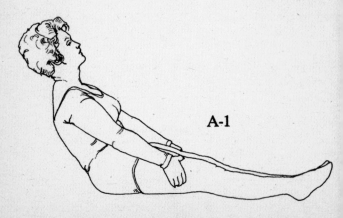

A-1

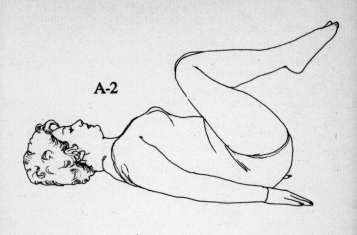

A-2

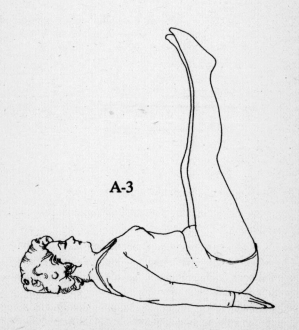

A-3

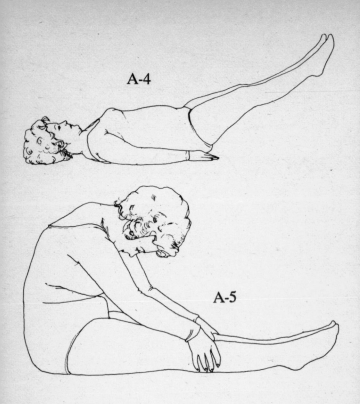

A-4

A-5

(B) Perform the identical movements of (A) 1-4.

*1. Stretch your arms outward and come into the upright position **without** the aid of your hands.*

2. Without pause reach forward and take hold of your ankles. Pull trunk down to the position illustrated. Without pause straighten to the upright position and repeat the entire routine.

Perform 5 times in continuous slow motion. Upon completion return to the upright seated position and relax.

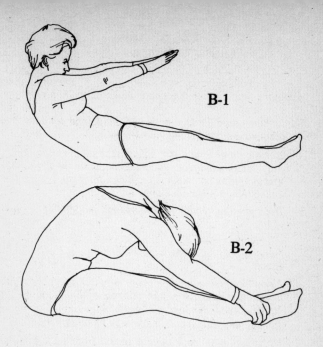

B-1

B-2

(C) *Perform the identical movements of (A) 1-4 and (B) 1.*

Now reach forward and hold your feet. Pull trunk down and bring your trunk and head into position illustrated.

Without pause straighten to the upright position and repeat the entire routine.

Perform 5 times in continuous slow motion. Upon completion return to the upright seated position and relax.

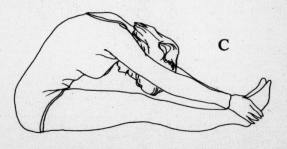

C

LEG CLASP
(To firm the thighs and calves)

Stand up gracefully from the previous seated position.

(A) 1. Place your heels together. Slowly bend forward and clasp your hands behind your knees.

2. Brace your hands firmly against the backs of the knees and very slowly draw your trunk down as far as possible without strain. Neck is relaxed and forehead is aimed at knees. (Knees must not bend.)

Hold your extreme position without motion for a count of 10.

(Remember that all "firming" exercises are held in the extreme positions. This is not a continuous motion exercise.)

Upon completion of the count of 10, relax your trunk and slowly return it to the position of Fig. 1. Keep the hands clasped. Pause several moments.

Repeat the forward pull of Fig. 2 and hold for 10, etc.

Perform the entire routine 5 times. Hold each extreme pull for 10.

Upon completion unclasp hands and very slowly raise your trunk to the upright position. Relax.

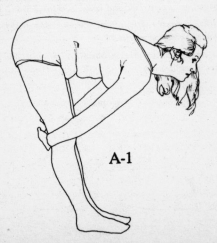

A-1

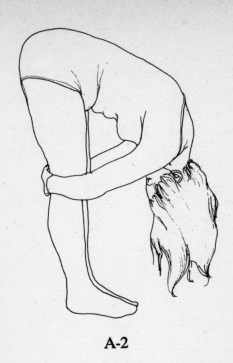

A-2

(B) *1. Now the hands are clasped behind the calves.*

2. Brace hands firmly against calves and very slowly draw your trunk down as far as possible without strain. Forehead should now be in position illustrated.

Hold your extreme position without motion for 10.

Raise your trunk several inches and relax for a moment but retain the clasp.

Repeat the pull. Perform the entire routine 5 times. Hold each extreme pull for 10.

Upon completion unclasp hands; very slowly raise your trunk to the upright position. Relax.

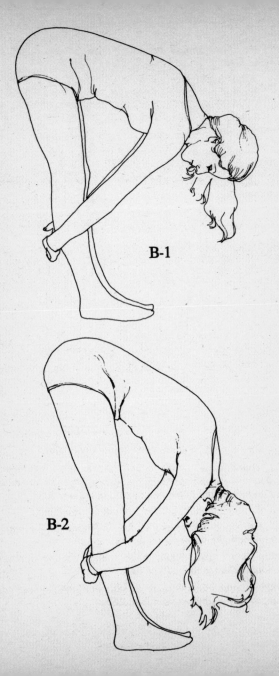

B-1

B-2

(C) Now you should be able to clasp your hands at the ankles.

Brace hands firmly against ankles and very slowly draw trunk down as far as possible without strain. You should now be able to bring your forehead very close to the knees.

Hold your extreme position without motion for 10.

Raise your trunk several inches and relax for a moment but retain the clasp.

Repeat and perform 5 times, holding each extreme pull for 10.

Very slowly raise your trunk to the upright position. Relax.

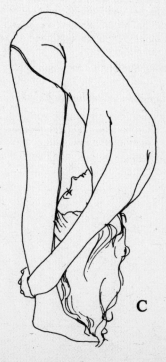

C

SIDE RAISE

(To firm the abdomen, arms, thighs and buttocks)

(A) *1. Lie down gracefully from the previous standing position and assume this position on your right side. Your legs are together and the right cheek rests in the right palm as illustrated. Place left hand firmly on floor.*

Push against floor with left hand and slowly raise left leg as high as possible. Hold your extreme position without motion for a count of 10.

Slowly lower leg to original position.

Repeat and perform 3 times.

2. Push as hard as possible against floor with left hand and raise both legs a short distance from the floor. Do not raise higher than illustrated. Legs must remain together and be raised straight up from the floor (they must not move behind or in front of your trunk). Hold as still as possible for 10.

Slowly lower the legs to the floor. Relax a moment and repeat.

Peform 3 times. Hold each raise for 10.

Following the final repetition, roll gracefully onto the left side. Perform the identical movements, raising the right leg as high as possible 3 times and both legs a short distance 3 times.

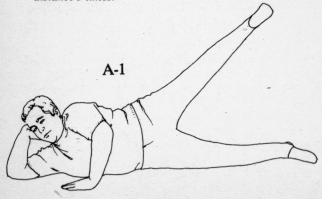

A-1

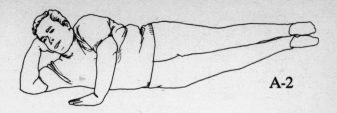

A-2

(B) Lie on your right side as depicted in (A).

Push as hard as possible against floor with your left hand and raise both legs an intermediate distance from the floor. This position is several inches higher than that of (A). Do not raise higher than illustrated. Legs must remain together and be raised straight up from the floor. Hold for 10.

Slowly lower legs to the floor. Relax a moment and repeat.

Perform 5 times. Hold each raise for 10.

Roll gracefully onto your left side. Perform the identical movements 5 times.

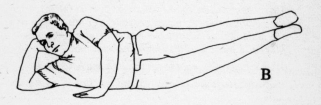

B

(C) Lie on your right side as depicted in (B).

Push as hard as possible against floor with your left hand; raise both legs as high as possible. This is the extreme position. Legs must remain together and be raised straight up from the floor. Hold for 10.

Slowly lower legs to the floor. Relax a moment and repeat.

Perform 5 times. Hold each raise for 10.

Roll gracefully onto your left side. Perform the identical movements 5 times.

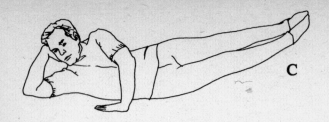

ABDOMINAL EXERCISES

(To stimulate organs of the viscera; to tone the
abdominal muscles; to reduce abdominal weight)

*(A) 1. Move gracefully into the cross-legged posture from
the previous lying position. Rest hands on knees.*

*Pull your abdomen in by contracting the muscles as
much as possible.*

*2. A closeup of the contraction. The degree of your con-
traction is unimportant in the beginning. One or two
inches will be adequate and effective. Hold the contraction for a count of 5.*

*Upon completion of the count of 5 attempt to "snap"
the abdomen out as far as possible. Do not simply relax
the abdomen or push it out but attempt a forceful snapping movement with the abdominal muscles.*

Without pause *repeat the contraction and hold for 5.*

*Perform 10 times. Relax. Stand up slowly and grace-
fully.*

*3. Execute the identical movements in this standing
position. Study the illustration. Knees bend slightly outward. Hands are placed firmly on the thighs with all
fingers, including thumb, pointing inward.*

*Perform 5 times. With each contraction push down hard
on the thighs. Hold each contraction for 5. Remember to
"snap" the abdomen out.*

Upon completion slowly straighten upright and relax.

*4. This is the All-Fours position. Legs are together,
palms firmly on floor, arms parallel with knees, head
lowered.*

Perform 5 times. Hold each contraction for 5.

Following the final repetition return to the cross-legged posture and relax.

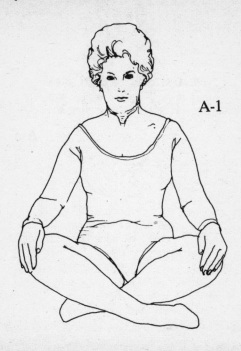

A-1

A-2

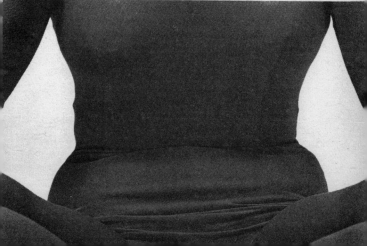

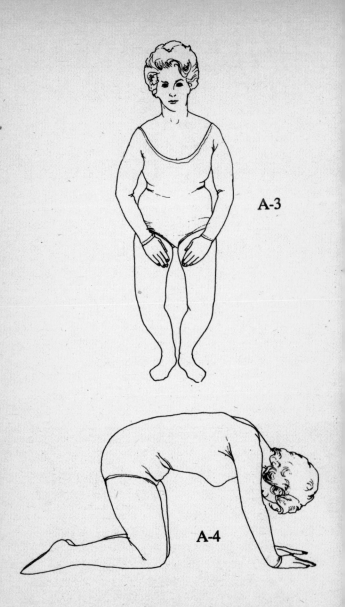

A-3

A-4

*(B) Sufficient abdominal weight has now been lost so that we may attempt a partial "lift" of the abdomen. It is essential to understand that this lifting movement can be successfully accomplished only if **all air is completely exhaled from your lungs and no air is allowed to enter while the movements are being performed.***

Exhale deeply and attempt a partial lift of the abdomen as illustrated. Hold the lift for a count of 2.

"Snap" the abdomen out as previously practiced

Without pause repeat the lifting and snapping out.

*With a little practice you will be able to perform 5 lifts to **each exhalation.** Do this 5 times so that you will have performed 25 movements in all.*

Relax upon completion. Stand up slowly and gracefully.

Refer to (A) 3. Perform 25 movements (5 lifts to each exhalation) in the standing position.

Refer to (A) 4. Perform 25 movements in the All-Fours position.

Following the final repetition return to the cross-legged posture and relax.

B

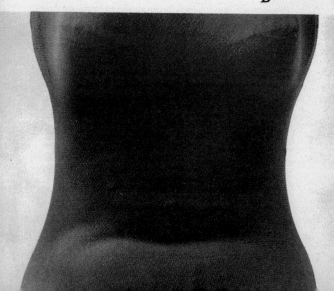

It is necessary to catch on to the knack of executing the movements **while the breath is exhaled.** All air must be expelled and kept out in order to create a vacuum or you will not be able to lift sufficiently to form the "hollow" as you see illustrated. We can further describe this movement as a "sucking in" of the abdomen, inward and upward. Imagine that you are attempting to breathe very deeply from the abdominal area. No air actually enters your lungs but the abdominal area goes through the motions of this deep breath during which it is sucked inward and upward.

Patient practice will be necessary to accomplish these highly rewarding movements. Once the lifting technique is mastered, there is no further need for the contractions.

You will be performing 75 movements in the entire exercise. Rest briefly between each group. Each lift is held for a count of 2 and there is no pause between the snapping-out movement and the next lift. An even, steady rhythm, not speed, is important.

(C) *Continued loss of weight now makes this extreme lifting movement possible.*

   As in (B) all air is completely exhaled and the identical movements are performed. However, you will note that the lift is deeper.

   Perform 25 movements in the seated posture (Half or Full Lotus) as described in (B).

   Perform 25 movements in the standing position.

   Perform 25 movements in the All-Fours position.

   Following the final repetition return to the cross-legged posture and relax.

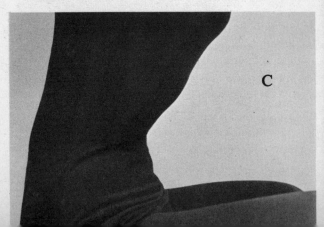

C

DIRECTION OF THE LIFE-FORCE

(To "recharge" the organism)

(A) 1. There is a storehouse of energy in the solar plexus. Our objective is to transfer this energy, or life-force, from the solar plexus to the forehead (the so-called "third eye" area) in order to raise the vibrations of the entire organism.

Lie down gracefully from the preceding exercise.

Close your eyes. Place the fingertips of both hands on your solar plexus.

Inhale a slow, quiet, deep breath. During the inhalation visualize in your mind's eye the life-force that is in the air you are breathing, passing through your nostrils and lungs and being drawn into your fingertips from the solar plexus. Attempt to visualize this life-force as a brilliant white light similar to that of sunlight.

2. Retain the air in your lungs. Hold the image of the white light (your mind must not wander).

With the breath retained, move your fingertips up to rest lightly on the forehead (the area between the eyebrows).

Now begin a slow, quiet, deep exhalation. During the exhalation direct the life-force (visualized as a brilliant white light) into your head. Gradually your entire head is flooded with the white light.

When the lungs are empty transfer the fingertips back to the solar plexus.

Without pause begin the next inhalation; retain the image of the white light being drawn into your fingertips and repeat the movements described above.

It is necessary to keep your mind clear of all extraneous thoughts during this exercise so that you can concentrate fully on the white light. Although the image of the white light may not be entirely clear or consistent in the beginning, this will come with subsequent practice.

Perform 7 times.

Upon completion rest your arms at your sides. Allow the body to become completely limp for several minutes.

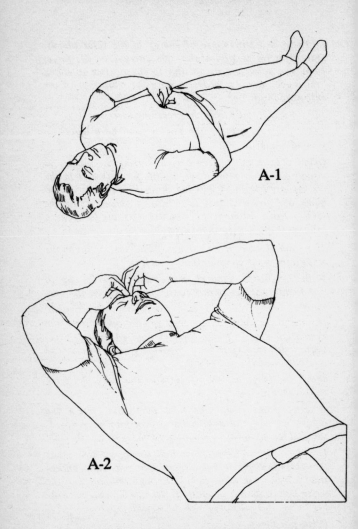

A-1

A-2

(B) & (C) The technique is identical with that of (A).

ROUTINE 2

COMPLETE BREATH

Begin today's routine by performing the Complete Breath 5 times, exactly as learned in Routine 1.

TRIANGLE

(To streamline the sides, waist and thighs)

(A) 1. Rise gracefully from the seated position of the Complete Breath and assume a stance with your legs approximately two feet apart.

Gracefully raise your arms to shoulder level.

2. Slowly bend to the left and place your left hand against the left knee or thigh. Note the position of the right arm.

3. Without pause, bend trunk to the left as illustrated. The right arm is now brought over the head so that it is parallel with the floor. Knees remain straight; neck is relaxed.

Without pause slowly straighten to the upright position of Fig. 1.

Without pause perform the identical movements by bending to the right.

Without pause straighten to the upright position and repeat the entire routine.

Perform 10 times in continuous slow motion. Upon completion, slowly and gracefully lower arms to sides; bring the feet together and relax.

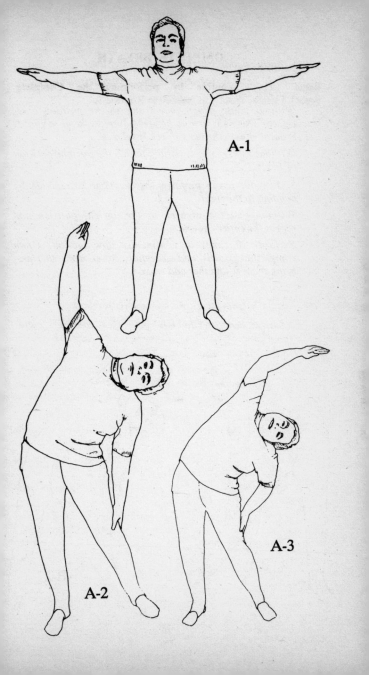

A-1

A-2

A-3

(B) 1. *Widen your stance (with relation to (A)1.)*

Gracefully raise your arms to shoulder level.

Slowly bend to the left and place your left hand against your left calf.

Without pause lower your trunk to the position illustrated. The right arm is brought over the head so that it is parallel with the floor. Neck is relaxed.

Without pause, slowly straighten to the upright position of Fig. 1.

2. Without pause perform the identical movements by bending to the right.

Without pause straighten to the upright position and repeat the entire routine.

Perform 10 times in continuous slow motion. Upon completion, slowly and gracefully lower arms to sides; bring the feet together and relax.

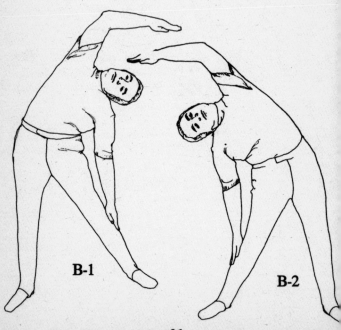

B-1   **B-2**

(C) *Assume the widest stance possible.*

Gracefully raise your arms to shoulder level.

Slowly bend to the left and place left hand against lower calf or ankle.

Without pause lower your trunk as far as possible. Right arm is brought over your head so that it is parallel with the floor.

Without pause, slowly straighten to the upright position of Fig. 1.

Without pause perform the identical movements by bending to the right.

Without pause straighten to the upright position and repeat the entire routine.

Perform 10 times in continuous slow motion. Upon completion, slowly and gracefully lower arms to sides; bring the feet together and relax.

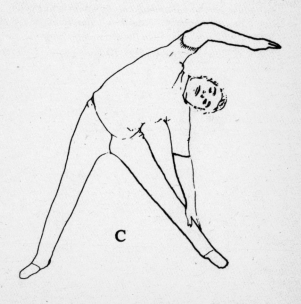

C

TWIST

(To trim inches from the waistline)

(A) 1. *Sit down gracefully; stretch your legs straight outward.*

Cross right leg over left with right knee raised as illustrated.

Place right hand firmly on the floor behind you for balance.

Hold your right knee firmly with left hand.

2. *Very slowly twist your head and trunk as far to the right as possible.*

Without pause return to the frontward position of Fig. 1. Do not release hold on leg.

Perform 10 times in continuous slow motion.

Upon completion stretch your right leg outward. Without pause perform the identical movements to the left 10 times in continuous slow motion. (Simply exchange the words "left" and "right" in the above directions.)

Upon completion stretch legs straight outward and relax.

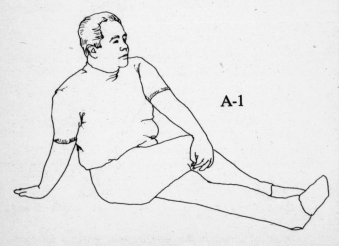

A-1

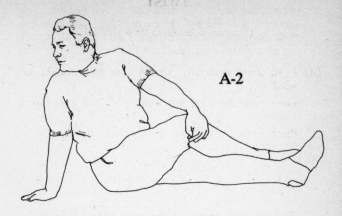

A-2

(B) 1. Sit with your legs outstretched. Take hold of your left foot and place it as illustrated. Heel is drawn in as far as possible.

2. Bring your right foot in and take hold of the ankle.

3. Swing the right leg over the left knee. Place the sole of the right foot firmly on the floor.

4. Place your right hand firmly on the floor behind you for balance.

5. Now bring your left arm over the right knee and brace your left elbow against the knee.

6. Very slowly twist your head and trunk to the **right**. Chin is close to the shoulder and trunk remains erect.

Without pause return to the frontward position of Fig. 5. Keep elbow braced against knee.

Without pause repeat the twist and perform 10 times in continuous slow motion.

Upon completion stretch both legs outward. Without pause perform the identical movements to the **left** 10 times in continuous slow motion. (Exchange the words "left" and "right" in the above directions.)

Upon completion stretch legs straight outward and relax.

In initial attempts this exercise may prove a bit complicated because of the hand and leg movements. However, it will be learned permanently after approximately three days of practice. This is a highly effective exercise and should not be neglected.

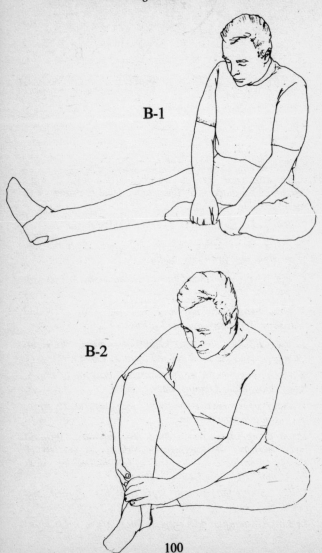

B-1

B-2

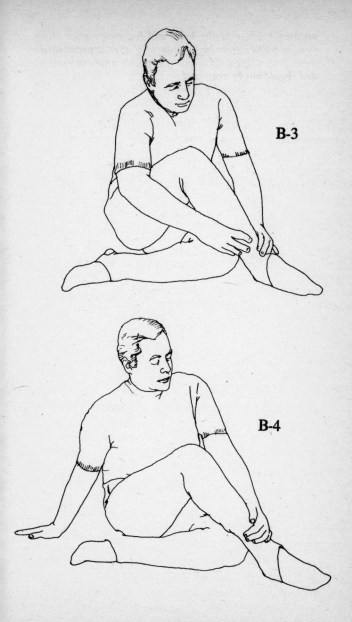

B-3

B-4

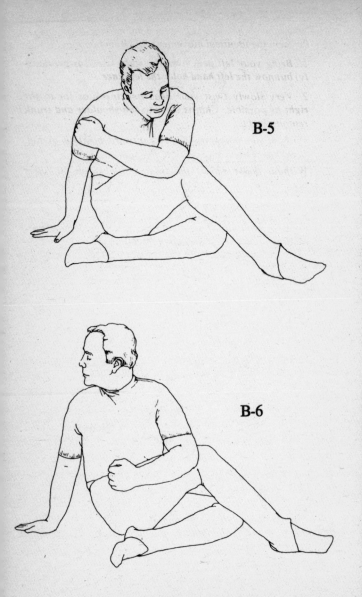

B-5

B-6

(C) *Perform the identical movements of (B) 1-4.*

*1. Bring your left arm over the right knee (as previously) but now the **left hand holds the left knee**.*

*2. Very slowly twist your head and trunk as far to the **right** as possible. Chin is close to the shoulder and trunk remains erect.*

Without pause return to the frontward position of Fig. 1. Do not release hold on knee.

Without pause repeat the twist and perform 10 times in continuous slow motion.

*Upon completion stretch both legs outward. Without pause perform the identical movements to the **left** 10 times in continuous slow motion. (Exchange the words "left" and "right" in the above directions.)*

Upon completion stretch legs straight outward and relax.

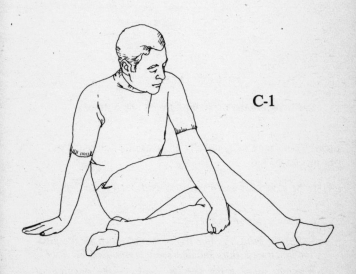

C-1

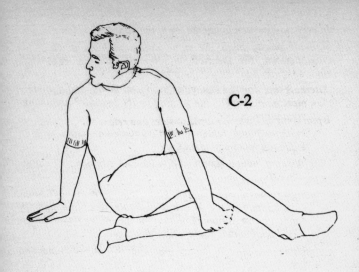

LEG OVER

(To reduce the waist, hips, thighs and buttocks)

Lower your trunk as gracefully as possible until your back is resting on the floor.

(A) 1. Stretch your arms outward and bring your left knee in.

2. Slowly straighten the leg.

3. Slowly bring the left leg over and down to the position illustrated. Both shoulders must remain on the floor.

Without pause bring the leg back to the position of Fig. 2.

In very slow motion lower the leg to the floor.

Without pause, bend the right knee and bring it in. Now perform the identical movements with the right leg.

Alternate the legs and perform 10 times in continuous slow motion.

Upon completion lower arms to sides and relax.

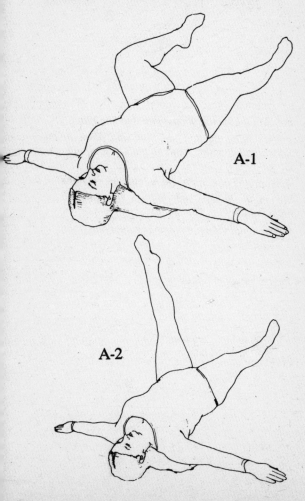

A-1

A-2

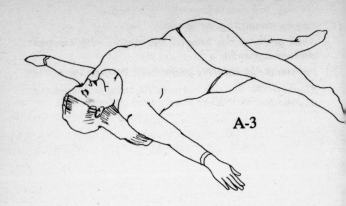

A-3

(B) Perform the identical movements of *(A)* 1 and 2.

Slowly bring the left leg over and down to touch the floor as illustrated. Both shoulders must remain on the floor.

Perform the identical movements with the right leg.

Alternate the legs and perform 10 times in continuous slow motion.

Upon completion lower arms to sides and relax.

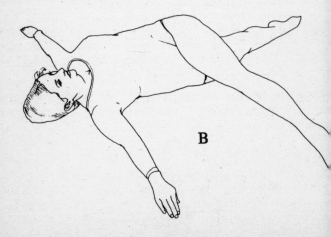

B

(C) *Perform the identical movements of (A) 1-2.*

Now, as the leg is lowered it is held as high toward the head as possible.

Perform the identical movements with the right leg.

Alternate the legs and perform 10 times in continuous slow motion.

Upon completion lower arms to sides and relax.

C

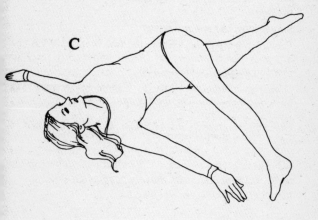

CHIN EXERCISE

(To reduce the chin(s)).

Raise the trunk and assume a cross-legged posture.

(A) 1. Relax your jaw.

2. Slowly raise the jaw so that the bottom teeth are placed over the upper teeth and you feel a tightening of the chin.

Slowly relax the jaw and repeat.

Perform 10 times in continuous slow motion. Relax for a few moments and repeat the 10 movements twice so that you do 30 movements in all.

(Thirty is minimum; 50 to 75 of these movements may be performed at various times of the day.)

(B) The chin movements are identical with those learned in (A).

(C) 1-2 The chin movements are identical with those learned in (A). (Compare (C) with those of (A) 1-2 and note lost of weight in this model's face.)

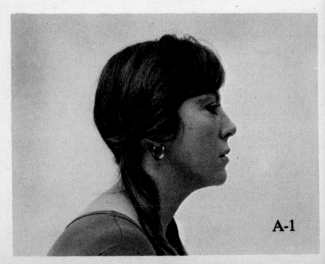

A-1

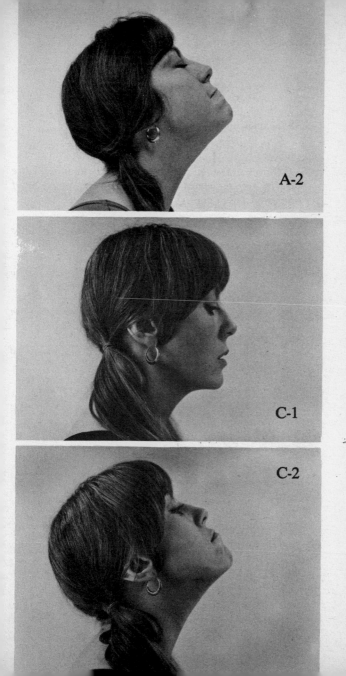

A-2

C-1

C-2

BACK STRETCH

(To firm the back and legs)

(A) 1. Sit with your legs outstretched, feet touching. **In** *very slow* **motion** *raise your arms and lean backward several inches (to tone the abdominal muscles).*

2. In very slow motion, with your arms outstretched, execute a forward "dive." Remember to perform your movements with the grace, poise and balance of a ballet dancer.

3. Take a firm grip of your upper calves, just below the knees.

4. Pull on your calves and, in very slow motion, lower the trunk as far as it will go without strain. Several inches is adequate in the beginning. Elbows must bend outward and head is down, neck relaxed. Hold without motion for 20. (Remember to count rhythmically, in approximate seconds.)

It is of no consequence how far down you are able to bring your trunk; only two inches is satisfactory. The essential thing is that you simply hold your extreme position without motion for the count of 20.

When the count of 20 is completed, in very slow motion straighten your trunk to an upright position and simultaneously raise your arms into the position of Fig. 1. Lean backward and repeat the movements.

Perform 5 times, holding each of the extreme positions for 20.

Upon completion slowly straighten to the upright position. Rest your hands on your knees and relax.

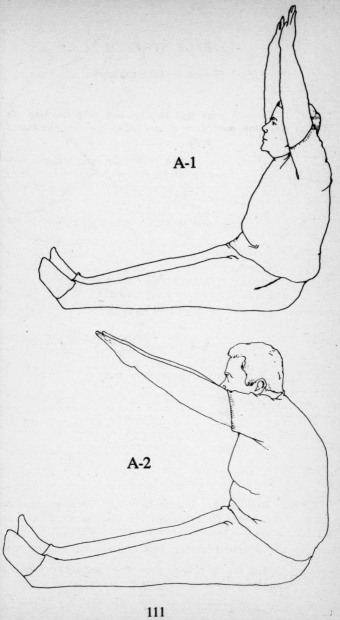

A-1

A-2

111

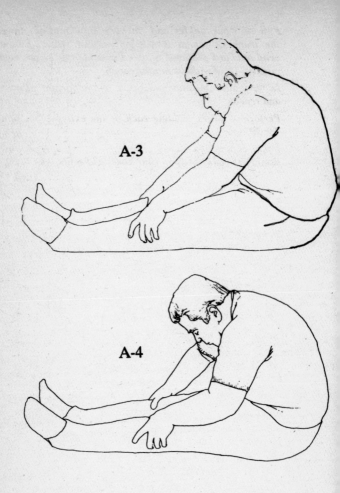

A-3

A-4

(B) 1. Refer to the movements of (A). These intermediate movements are essentially the same, although now we attempt to bend farther in both directions.

Bend several inches farther backward as depicted.

2. Execute the slow-motion "dive" and take a firm grip on the lower calves or, if possible, the ankles.

Pull on your ankles and, in very slow motion, lower the trunk as far as it will go without strain. Elbows bend outward and head is aimed toward your knees, neck relaxed. Hold without motion for 20.

In very slow motion straighten to an upright position and repeat.

Perform 5 times, holding each of the extreme positions for 20.

Upon completion slowly straighten to the upright position. Rest your hands on your knees and relax.

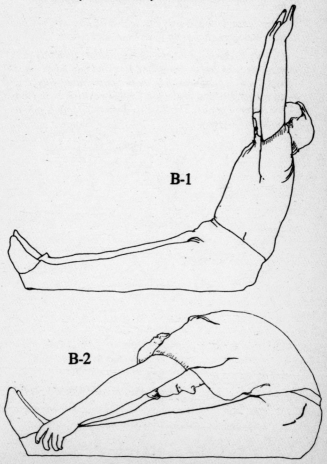

B-1

B-2

(C) 1. Perform the movements of (B) 1.

Execute the slow-motion "dive" forward. If you will "rock" or "sway" very gently from side to side as you bend forward, you will help to loosen your spine.

Take a firm hold on your feet.

2. Pull your trunk slowly downward and attempt to rest your forehead on your knees. Hold without motion for 20.

Perform 5 times, holding each of the extreme positions for 20.

Upon completion slowly straighten to the upright position. Rest your hands on your knees and relax.

3. This is the most advanced position. It provides maximum firming for the back and legs and can be attempted after you are comfortable in the position of Fig. 2 and no longer find it a challenge. In this position both elbows are lowered toward the floor as depicted. Hold for 20 and perform 3 times.

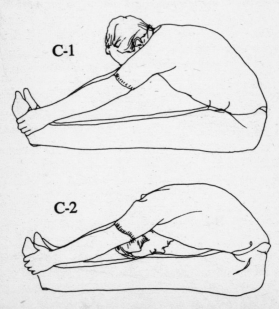

C-1

C-2

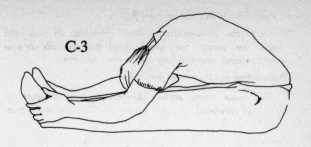

C-3

SHOULDER RAISE

(To firm the arms, chest and bust)

(A) 1. Seated in a simple cross-legged posture interlace your fingers behind your back.

2. In very slow motion raise your arms to approximately the position illustrated. Hold motionless for a count of 10.

Slowly lower your arms to the position of Fig. 1 and without pause repeat.

Perform 5 times and hold each extreme position for 10.

Upon completion unclasp your hands, rest them on your knees and relax.

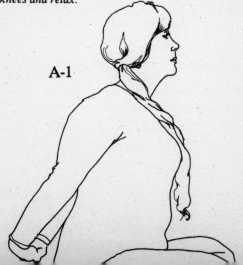

A-1

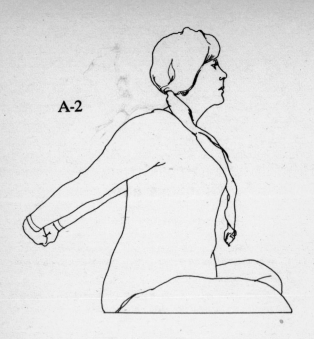

A-2

(B) You can now assume a Half-Lotus posture.

Loss of weight in your arms should now enable you to raise them to approximately the position illustrated. Hold motionless for a count of 10.

Slowly lower the arms and without pause repeat.

Perform 5 times; hold each extreme position for 10.

Upon completion unclasp your hands, rest them on your knees and relax.

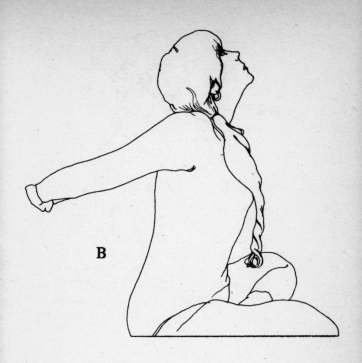

B

(C) *Sit in either the Half or Full-Lotus.*

Continued loss of weight in your arms should now enable you to raise them to approximately this position. Hold motionless for a count of 10.

Slowly lower the arms and without pause repeat.

Perform 5 times; hold each extreme position for 10.

Upon completion unclasp your hands, rest them on your knees and relax.

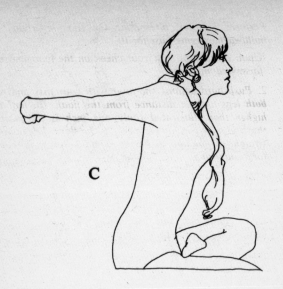

C

LOCUST

(To firm the abdomen, hips, buttocks, legs and arms)

(A) 1. From the previous seated position move gracefully into a lying position with your chin resting on the floor.

Make fists of your hands and place them thumbs down firmly on the floor at your sides.

Push against the floor with your fists and very slowly raise your left leg as high as possible. Knee is as straight as possible. Hold motionless for 10.

Very slowly lower the left leg to the floor and, without pause, perform the identical movements with the right leg.

Perform 3 times, alternating the legs (left-right) and hold each extreme raise for 10.

Upon completion rest your cheek on the floor and relax for several moments.

2. **Push** hard against the floor with your fists and raise **both** legs a short distance from the floor. Do not raise higher than illustrated (only one inch is adequate in the beginning). Chin remains on the floor, knees are as straight as possible. Hold the raised position motionless for a count of 5.

Very slowly lower legs to the floor. Relax a moment and repeat.

Perform 3 times; hold each raise for 5.

Upon completion rest your cheek on the floor and allow all muscles to relax.

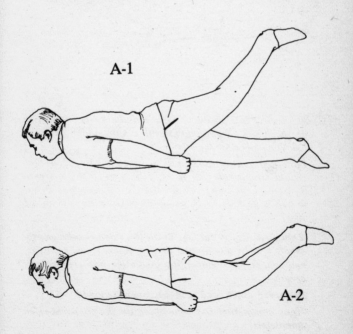

A-1

A-2

119

(B) Increased muscle tone should now enable you to raise the legs to this higher position. Legs are together and knees remain as straight as possible. Do not raise higher than illustrated. Hold as steady as possible for a count of 10.

Very slowly lower legs to the floor. Relax a moment and repeat.

Perform 3 times; hold each raise for 10.

Upon completion rest your cheek on the floor and relax completely.

B

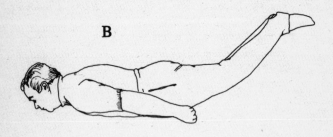

*(C) In the starting position (with your chin, legs and fists on the floor) fill your lungs with a slow, quiet, deep inhalation and **retain the breath.***

Increased muscle tone and significant loss of weight should now enable you to raise the legs to this extreme position. Legs must remain together, knees may bend, breath is held. Hold as steady as possible for a count of 10.

*Very slowly lower the legs to the floor and **simultaneously** exhale slowly, quietly and deeply. Relax a few moments and repeat. (Remember the inhalation and retention of breath.)*

Perform 3 times; hold each extreme raise for 10.

Upon completion rest your cheek on the floor and relax completely.

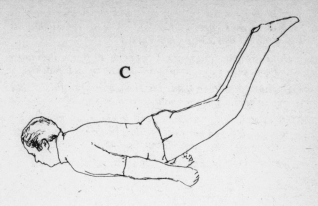

C

HEAD STAND

(For the health of the entire organism, with emphasis
on promoting good blood circulation as an aid in
weight regulation)

*(A) 1. Move gracefully into a seated posture from the pre-
vious lying position. Place a pillow (which you should
have on hand for this exercise) on your mat.*

Sit on your heels.

*Interlace your fingers; bend forward and place your
hands and arms on the pillow as illustrated.*

*2. Rest the top of your head on the pillow; the back
of your head is cradled firmly in your hands.*

*3. Place your toes on the floor and push up so that your
body forms an arch.*

4. Walk forward on your toes and move your knees as close to your chest as possible. (Knees bend slightly as you move them toward your chest.)

*Hold without motion for a count of 10 in the beginning and **gradually** add seconds until a count of 30 is reached.*

Do not go farther than this elementary position of the Head Stand and do not hold more than 30.

Upon completion of the count, lower your knees to the floor so that you are back in the position of Fig. 2. Rest in this position for an additional count of 20-30 seconds.

Slowly raise your head and relax in a seated posture.

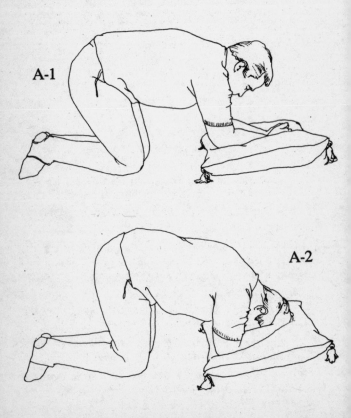

A-1

A-2

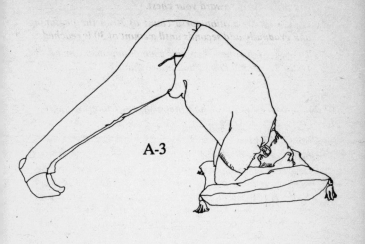

A-3

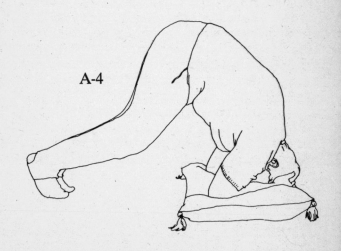

A-4

(B) Sufficient weight has now been lost so that we execute this intermediate position.

Refer to (A) 1-4.

*Push off from the floor lightly with your toes and transfer your weight so that it is evenly distributed between your head and forearms. This is the second stage of the Head Stand. Do not attempt to straighten your legs at this time. Hold for a count of 10 in the beginning and **gradually** add seconds until a count of 60 (one minute) is reached.*

Bringing your knees as close to the chest as possible (A) 4 will enable you to transfer your balance more easily. If you lose your balance attempt the posture three times, then try again on the following day. If you continue to roll forward you may use a wall for support by placing your pillow about six inches from the wall before beginning.

Very slowly, with complete control, lower your feet and knees to the floor (see (A) 2). Do not allow the feet to "bang" against the floor. Remain with your head down for a count of 30-60 seconds.

Slowly raise your head and relax in a seated posture.

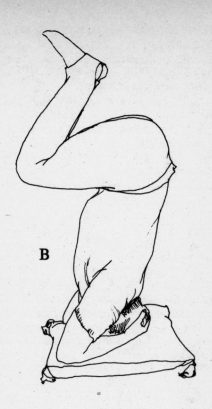

B

(C) 1. Continued loss of weight will enable us to perfect the completed posture.

Refer to (A) 1-4 and (B) 1.

Very slowly begin to straighten your legs. Remain in this position with as little movement as possible for a count of 10 to make certain that you are secure and well balanced. If you are shaky, do not continue upward. Practice to gain steadiness in this position before going on.

2. The completed posture. The entire body is as straight

as possible. Hold for a count of 10 in the beginning and gradually add seconds over a period of several months until approximately three minutes are reached. You may place a clock to the side of your head so that you can time the extreme position.

Come out of the posture smoothly and gracefully by lowering your knees slowly to your chest and then lowering your feet to the floor. Remain with your head down for a count of 30-60 seconds.

Slowly *raise your head and relax in a seated posture.*

C-1

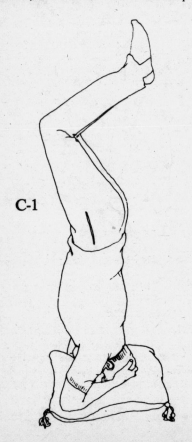

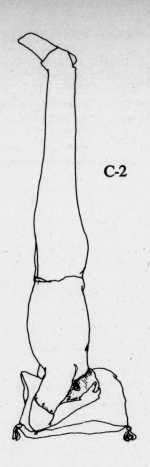

C-2

ALTERNATE NOSTRIL BREATHING

(To maintain equanimity)

This exercise is scheduled to terminate each third day of practice. However, because of its excellent effect on quelling the desires of the "compulsive" eater, it may be used whenever necessary. When the unnatural craving for food arises, the student can seclude himself and perform several rounds of this breathing exercise. The soothing state of consciousness that results will usually dispel the need to eat.

(A) 1. Study the illustration and place your right hand as depicted. The index and middle fingers rest lightly between the eyebrows. The thumb rests lightly against the right nostril and the ring finger is against the left. Eyes are closed.

Execute a deep, slow, quiet exhalation through both nostrils.

2. Begin a rhythmic beat in your mind.

Press the thumb against the right nostril to close it tightly.

Execute a deep, slow, quiet inhalation through your left nostril during a rhythmic count of 8 beats.

3. Keep the rhythmic beat going.

Press the left nostril closed with your ring finger so that both nostrils are now closed. Without missing a beat retain the air in your lungs for a count of 4.

4. Keep the rhythmic beat going.

Release the thumb slightly so that the right nostril is open. Keep the left closed. Without missing a beat execute a deep, slow, quiet exhalation through the right nostril in a count of 8.

Keep the rhythmic beat going.

Keep the left nostril closed. When the deep exhalation is completed, without pause begin a deep, slow, quiet inhalation through the right nostril in a count of 8.

Keep the rhythmic beat going.

Close the right nostril (both nostrils are now closed) and retain the air in your lungs for a count of 4.

Keep the rhythmic beat going.

*Open the **left** nostril (the right remains closed) and execute a deep, slow, quiet exhalation through the left nostril in a count of 8.*

Keep the rhythmic beat going.

*Keep the right nostril closed. When the exhalation is completed you have returned to the original starting point and this completes **one round** of the exercise.*

Without pause begin the next round by executing a deep, slow, quiet inhalation through the left nostril in a count of 8.

Continue the procedure as described above.

Here is a summary of the exercise:

inhale through the left	*— count 8*
close both nostrils and retain	*— count 4*
exhale through the right	*— count 8*
inhale through the right	*— count 8*
close both nostrils and retain	*— count 4*
exhale through the left	*— count 8*

begin again, i.e. inhale through the left, etc.

Perform 5 complete rounds without pause.

A cross-legged posture should be assumed; eyes are lowered (or closed); counting is rhythmic and exact. (The steady rhythm is very important in this exercise to accomplish the "stabilizing.")

Upon completion rest your hands on your knees and relax completely. You will experience a very elevated state of consciousness. Sit quietly (with eyelids lowered) for several minutes.

129

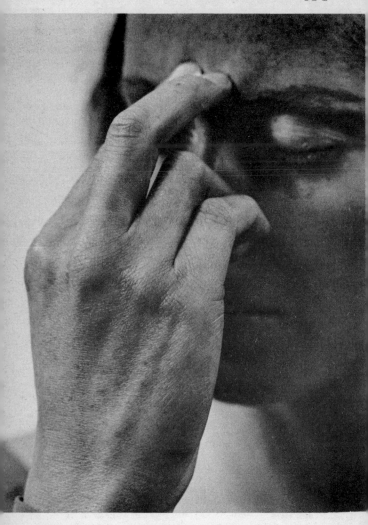

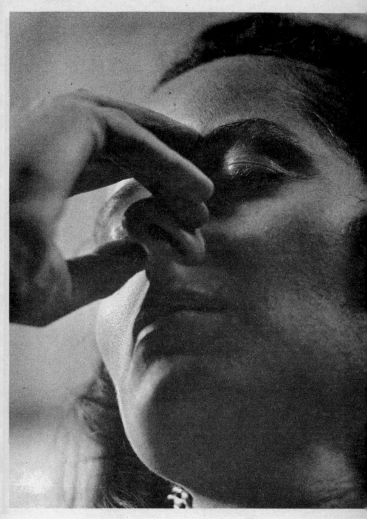

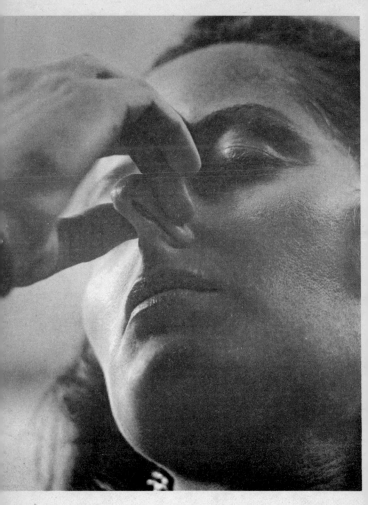

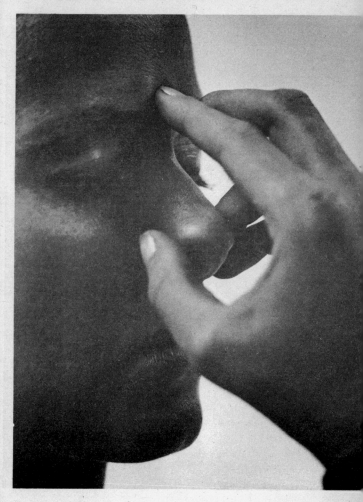

(B) & (C) The technique is identical with that of (A) except that the Half or Full-Lotus could now be assumed.

ROUTINE 3

COMPLETE BREATH

Begin today's routine by performing the Complete Breath 5 times, exactly as learned in Routine 1.

RISHI'S POSTURE

(To streamline the waist, hips and thighs)

Rise gracefully from the seated posture of the Complete Breath and assume a stance with heels together and arms at sides.

(A) 1. Slowly and gracefully raise your arms so that the hands meet in front at eye level.

2. Fix your gaze on the back of the hands and very slowly turn to the left.

3. Continue the twisting movement until a 90 degree position is reached.

4. Study the illustration. The right hand moves slowly down the right leg and holds the right knee firmly. The left hand moves behind you and your gaze follows the left hand.

5. The left arm has moved to the overhead position and your gaze is fixed on the back of the left hand.

Without pause very slowly raise your trunk back into the upright position and bring your arms back into the position of Fig. 1.

*Without pause begin to turn slowly to the **right**, then perform the identical movements, exchanging the words "right" and "left" in the above directions.*

Alternate the sides and perform 10 times in continuous slow motion.

Upon completion return to the frontward position of Fig. 1, gracefully lower arms to the sides and relax.

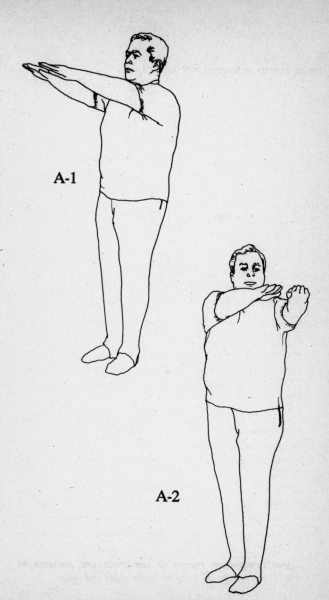

A-1

A-2

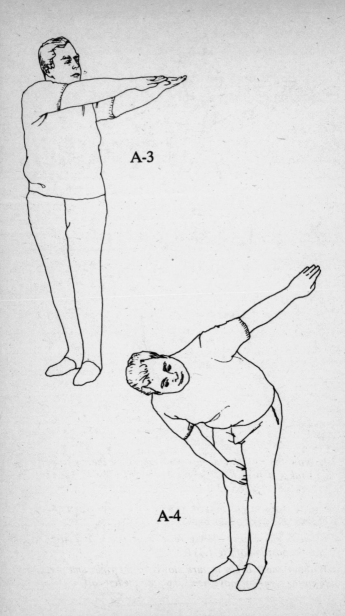

A-3

A-4

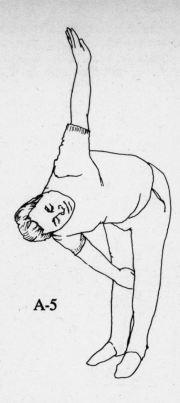

A-5

(B) Perform the movements of (A) 1-3.

*1. Now the right hand moves slowly down the right leg and takes a firm hold on the right **calf**. The left hand moves behind you as illustrated.*

2. The left arm has moved to the overhead position and your gaze is fixed on the back of the left hand.

Without pause very slowly raise your trunk and arms into the position of Fig. (A) 1.

*Without pause begin to turn slowly to the right and perform the identical movements, holding the **left** calf.*

Alternate the sides and perform 10 times in continuous slow motion.

Upon completion return to the frontward position of Fig. (A) 1, gracefully lower arms to the sides and relax.

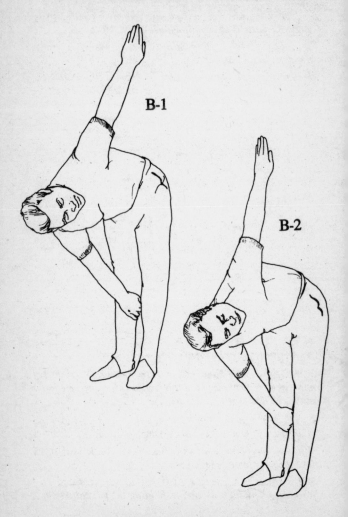

B-1

B-2

(C) *Perform the movements of (A) 1-3.*

*1. Now the right hand moves slowly down the right leg and takes a firm hold on the right **ankle**. The left hand moves behind you as illustrated.*

2. The left arm has moved into the overhead position and your gaze is fixed on the back of the left hand.

Without pause very slowly raise your trunk and arms into the position of Fig. (A) 1.

*Without pause begin to turn slowly to the **right** and perform the identical movements, holding the **left** ankle.*

Alternate the sides and perform 10 times in continuous slow motion.

Upon completion return to the frontward position of Fig. (A) 1, gracefully lower arms to the sides and relax.

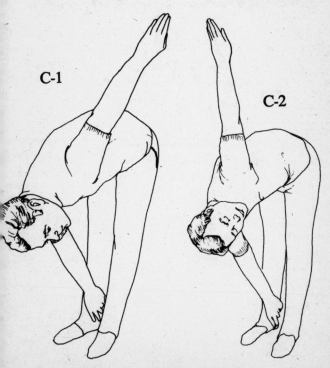

C-1

C-2

141

DANCER'S POSTURE

(To reduce the thighs and calves)

(A) 1. *Remain in the standing position with your heels together. Rest your hands on your head as illustrated. Palms are pressed firmly together.*

2. *In very slow motion bend your knees and lower your body into the position illustrated. Do not lower farther.*

3. *Without pause, in very slow motion, raise slowly to the upright position and come up high on toes.*

Without pause lower soles of feet to floor and perform 10 times in very slow motion.

Upon completion lower arms gracefully to the sides and relax.

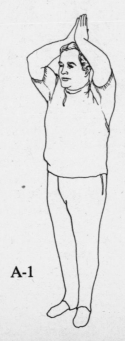

A-1

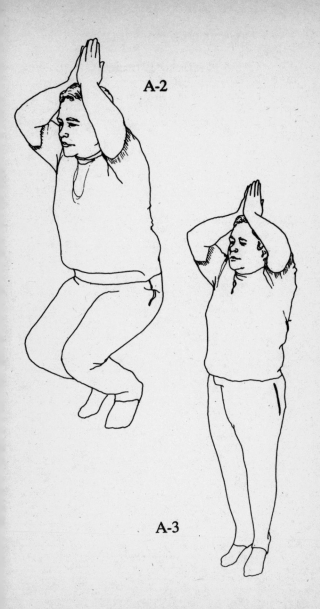

A-2

A-3

(B) In very slow motion the body is now lowered until buttocks touch heels. Knees remain close together.

Without pause, in very slow motion, raise slowly to the upright position and come up high on toes.

Without pause repeat and perform 10 times in very slow motion.

Upon completion lower arms gracefully to the sides and relax.

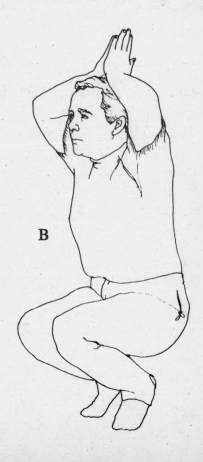

B

(C) The movements are identical- with those of (B). Continued loss of weight makes an even further lowering possible.

Perform 10 times.

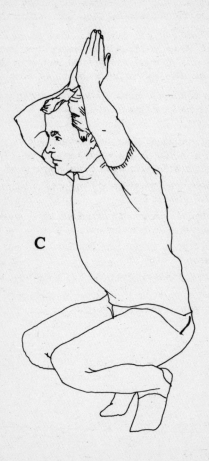

C

ROLL TWIST
(To reduce the waist and hips)

(A) *1. In a standing position, with your heels together, place your hands on your hips and bend forward several inches. Do not bend farther than illustrated. We now wish to roll and twist the trunk in a small circle.*

2. Slowly roll and twist your trunk to the left. Do not simply bend to the left but make certain to roll and twist with as much exaggerated motion in the waist as possible. Do not bend farther than illustrated.

3. In continuous slow motion roll and twist the trunk to the backward position. Do not go back farther than illustrated.

4. In continuous slow motion, and with the same exaggerated motion in the waist, roll and twist to the right. Remember that your trunk is outlining a small circle.

In continuous slow motion roll and twist to the frontward position of Fig. 1.

Perform 5 circles in continuous slow motion with a maximum of exaggerated waist motion.

Straighten to an upright position and relax for a few moments.

Perform 5 additional circles by moving first to the right.

Upon completion, straighten to the upright position, lower arms to the sides and relax.

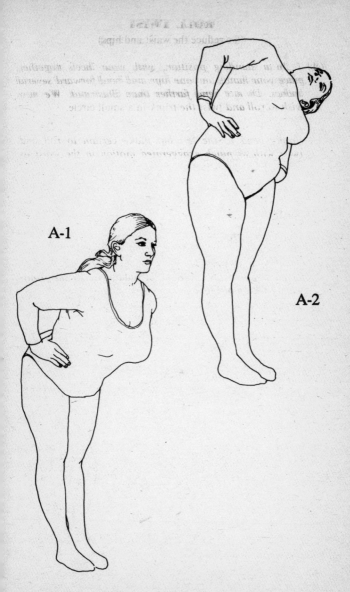

A-1

A-2

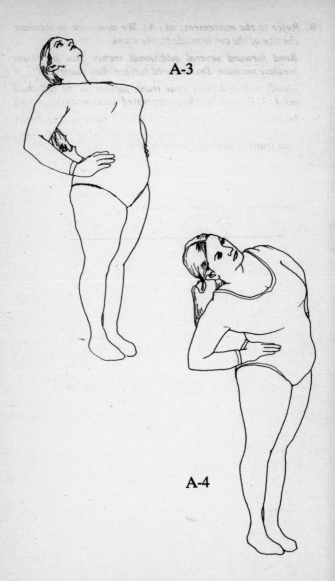

A-3

A-4

(B) Refer to the movements of (A). We now wish to increase the size of the circle made by the trunk.

Bend forward several additional inches into an intermediate position. Do not bend farther than illustrated.

Slowly roll and twist your trunk farther to the left than in (A) 2. Remember the exaggerated waist motion.

In continuous slow motion roll and twist to the backward, right and frontward positions. Remember that your trunk is outlining an intermediate circle.

In continuous slow motion perform 5 counter-clockwise circles and 5 clockwise circles.

Upon completion, straighten to the upright position, lower arms to the sides and relax.

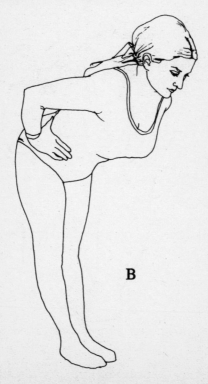

B

(C) 1. Refer to the movements of (A) and (B). We now wish to make the widest circle possible.

Bend forward to this extreme position.

2. Slowly roll and twist your trunk as far to the left as possible. Remember the exaggerated waist motion.

In continuous slow motion roll and twist to the extreme backward, right and frontward positions.

In continuous slow motion perform 5 counter-clockwise circles and 5 clockwise circles.

Upon completion, straighten to the upright position, lower arms to the sides and relax.

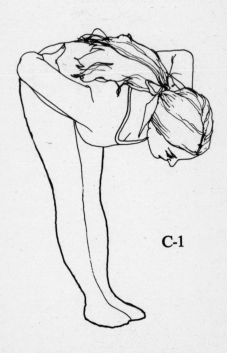

C-1

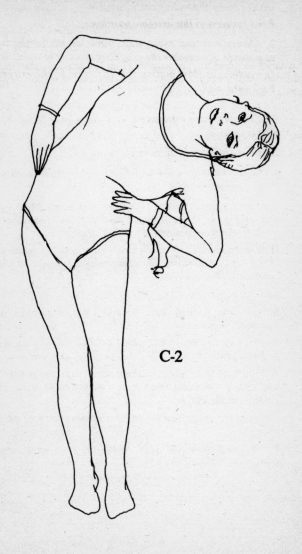

C-2

SEATED SIDE BEND

(To trim inches from waist and trunk)

Sit down as gracefully as possible from the previous standing position and assume a cross-legged posture. A pillow may prove helpful in this exercise.

(A) 1. Raise your arms gracefully and clasp your hands behind your head.

2. Slowly twist as far as possible to the left.

3. Slowly bend forward and bring right elbow as close to left knee as possible.

4. Without pause slowly straighten to the upright position of Fig. 1. Without pause slowly lower right elbow as far to the floor as possible without strain.

Without pause slowly straighten to the upright position of Fig. 1 and perform the identical movements to the opposite sides as follows:

Slowly twist as far as possible to the right.

Slowly bend forward and bring left elbow as close to right knee as possible.

Without pause slowly straighten to the upright position and now lower left elbow as far to the floor as possible.

Without pause slowly straighten to the upright position and repeat the entire routine, i.e., slowly twist as far as possible to the left, etc.

Perform the entire routine in continuous slow motion 7 times.

Upon completion rest your hands on your knees and relax.

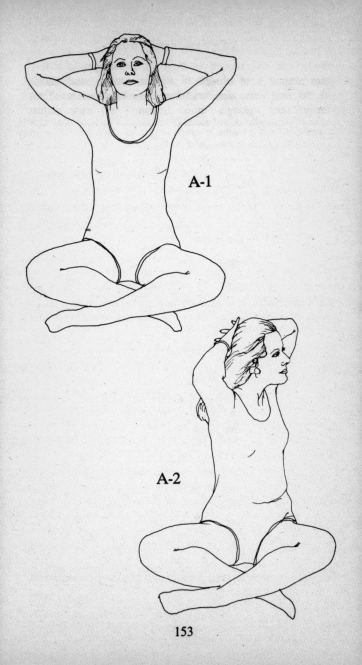

A-1

A-2

153

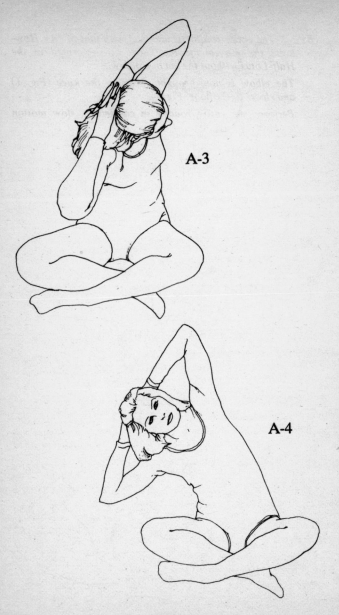

A-3

A-4

(B) 1-2 *The entire routine is identical with that of (A). However, the movements may now be performed in the Half-Lotus without the aid of a pillow.*

The elbow is now brought closer to the knee (Fig. 1) and closer to the floor (Fig. 2).

Perform the entire routine in continuous slow motion 7 times.

B-1

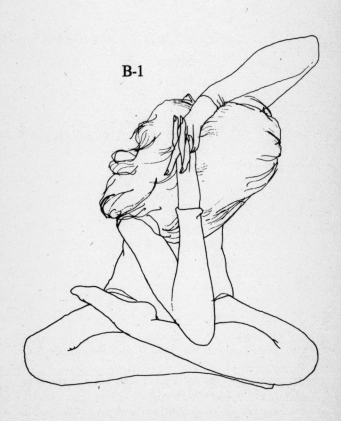

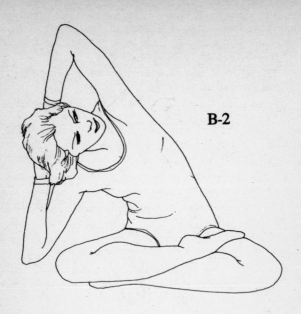

B-2

*(C) 1-2 The entire routine is identical with that of (B). How-
ever, the movements may now be performed in the Half
or Full-Lotus.*

*The elbow can now be brought very close to the knee
(Fig. 1) and to touch the floor (Fig. 2).*

*Perform the entire routine in continuous slow motion
7 times.*

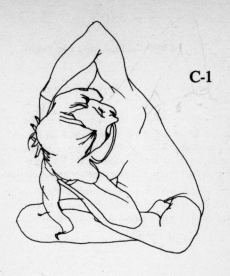

C-1

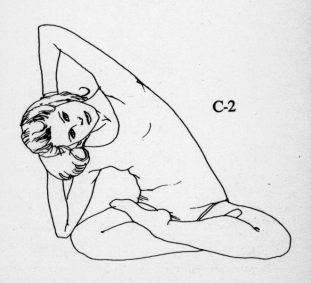

C-2

LION

(To firm the face, chin and neck)

(A) *1. Sit in the simple cross-legged posture. Rest hands on knees.*

2. Tense all muscles. Move trunk forward. Widen eyes, spread fingers. Extend your tongue as far out and down as possible. This is a very intensive movement and you must feel all of your neck muscles working. Hold without motion for 20. Do not relax the tongue during the hold.

Very slowly withdraw your tongue. Relax all muscles and relax for a few moments. Repeat and perform 5 times; hold each extreme position for 20.

A-1

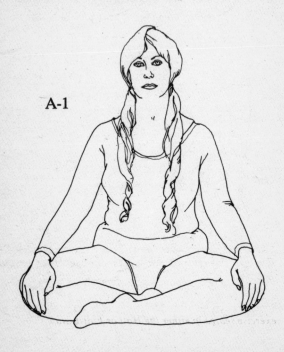

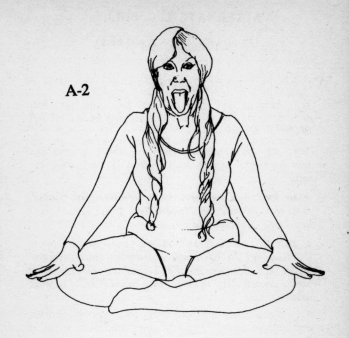

A-2

(B) The movements and repetitions are identical with (A). Perform the exercise seated in either the Half or Full-Lotus.

(C) The movements are identical with (A). Perform the exercise seated in either the Half or Full-Lotus.

ALTERNATE LEG PULL

(To firm the legs)

(A) 1. *Sit with your legs outstretched.*

Take hold of your right foot and place the right heel as illustrated. The sole rests against (not under) the left thigh.

2. In very slow motion raise your arms overhead and lean backward several inches. Head is back, look upward.

3. In very slow motion, with your arms outstretched, execute a forward bend and take a firm grip on your upper calf just below the knee.

4. Pull on your calf and, in very slow motion, lower the trunk as far as it will go without strain. Several inches is adequate in the beginning. Elbows must bend outward, head is down, neck relaxed. Hold without motion for 20.

Very slowly straighten your trunk to an upright position and simultaneously raise your arms into the position of Fig. 2. Lean backward and repeat the movements.

Perform 3 times, holding each stretch for 20.

Slowly straighten upright. Straighten your right leg. Rest your hands on your knees and relax a few moments.

Now perform the identical movements with the **right** *leg outstretched. Exchange the words "right" and "left" in the above directions.*

Perform 3 times with the right leg, holding each stretch for 20.

Upon completion slowly straighten to the upright position. Rest your hands on your knees and relax.

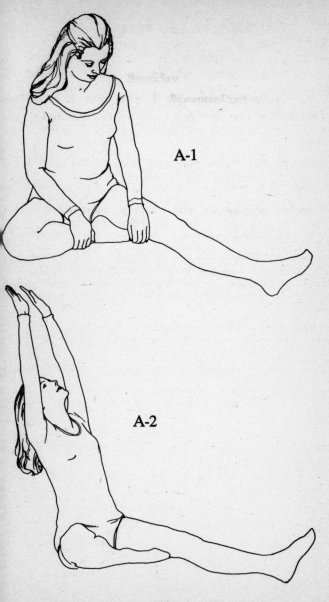

A-1

A-2

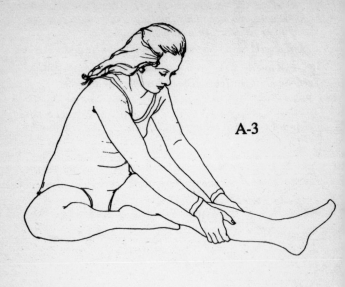

A-3

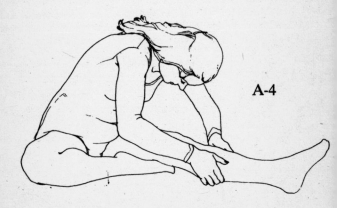

A-4

(B) 1. *Refer to the movements of (A). These intermediate movements are essentially the same although now we attempt to bend farther in both directions.*

Bend several inches farther backward as illustrated.

2. Execute the slow motion forward bend and take a firm grip on the lower left calf or, if possible, the ankle.

Pull on your left ankle and, in very slow motion, lower the trunk as far as it will go without strain. Elbows bend outward and head is aimed at left knee. Neck is relaxed. Hold for 20.

Very slowly straighten your trunk to an upright position and simultaneously raise your arms. Lean backward as in Fig. 1 and repeat the movements.

Perform 3 times, holding each stretch for 20.

Slowly straighten upright. Straighten your right leg. Rest your hands on your knees and relax a few moments.

*Perform the identical movements 3 times with the **right** leg outstretched; hold each stretch for 20.*

Relax upon completion.

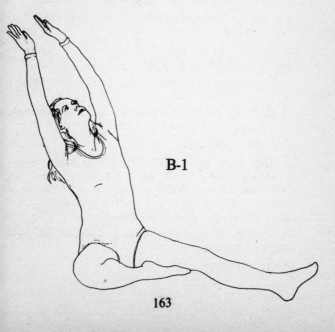

B-1

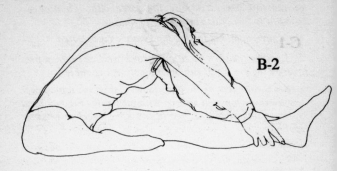

B-2

(C) 1. Perform the movements of (B) 1.

Execute the slow-motion forward bend and take a firm grip on your left foot.

2. Pull on your left foot and attempt to rest your forehead on the left knee. Hold for 20.

Perform 3 times, holding each of the extreme positions for 20.

*Perform the identical movements 3 times with the **right** leg outstretched; hold each stretch for 20.*

Relax upon completion.

3. This is the most advanced position that provides maximum firming for the leg. It can be attempted only after you are comfortable in the position of Fig. 2. In this position both elbows are lowered to touch the floor. Hold for 20 and perform 3 times.

Perform the identical movements 3 times with the right leg; hold each stretch for 20.

Relax upon completion.

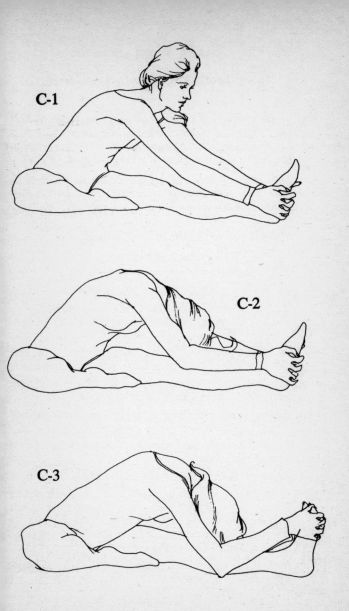

C-1

C-2

C-3

BACK PUSH-UP

(To firm the abdomen, legs, buttocks and arms)

(A) 1. *Move gracefully onto your back from the previous seated position. Bend your knees and bring your feet in as far as possible. Place the hands as illustrated. Note that the fingers are together and they point behind you.*

2. *Push your hands and feet against the floor and slowly raise your trunk a moderate distance only. Do not raise higher than illustrated. Knees are together. Hold for 10.*

Slowly lower the trunk to the floor. Repeat.

Perform 5 times, holding each raise for 10.

Upon completion lower arms and legs and relax.

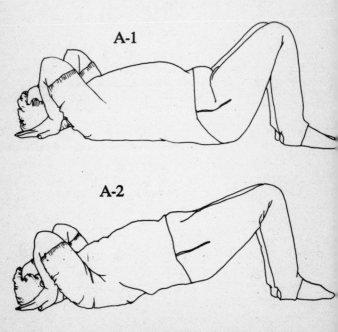

A-1

A-2

(B) Raise your trunk as high as possible. Knees remain together. Hold for 10.

Perform 5 times; hold each raise for 10.

Upon completion lower arms and legs and relax.

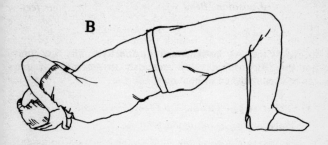

(C) Now we execute an advanced position. As the trunk is raised place the top of your head on the floor. Continue to push up as high as possible. Knees remain together. Hold for 10.

Perform 5 times; hold each raise for 10.

Upon completion lower arms and legs and relax.

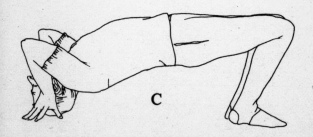

SHOULDER STAND

(For stimulation of the thyroid gland as an important
factor in weight control)

Persons who are more than 15 pounds overweight should
utilize the wall as an aid for the first stage of this posture.
If you are less than 15 pounds overweight, you may be able
to bypass the (A) positions and go directly to (B). You may
test the (B) positions very cautiously to determine if they
can be accomplished without discomfort.

*(A) 1. Place a **small** pillow 2 to 3 feet from a wall.*

*Place your right side **against** the wall.*

*Slowly turn toward the wall; swing your legs up against
the wall; lower your trunk so that your head and neck
rest on the pillow.*

*2. Brace your hands against your hips. Slowly "walk" up
the wall until your legs are as straight as possible.*

*Hold for 1 minute in the beginning and **gradually** add
seconds until 5 minutes are reached. Place a clock near
by.*

*To come out of the posture simply lower your feet to
the floor and then turn your body so that you can rest
your legs on the floor. Relax in a lying position for approximately 1 minute.*

This is a very important posture.

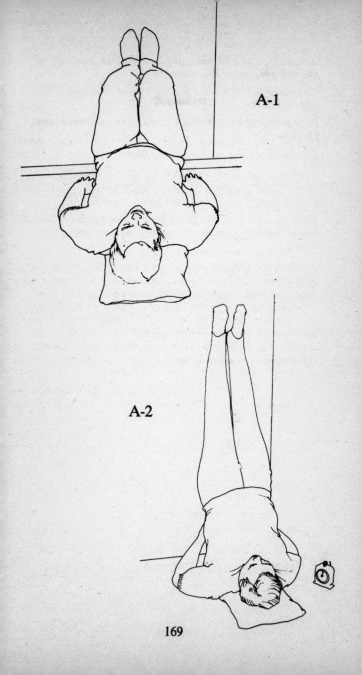

A-1

A-2

169

(B) *1. Sufficient weight has now been lost so that aid of the wall is no longer necessary.*

Place your palms against the floor; tense your abdominal and leg muscles.

Push palms against the floor and slowly raise your legs; knees are straight.

2. Swing your legs back over your head.

3. Brace your hands against your hips for support and very slowly straighten to a moderate upright position as illustrated. Do not straighten farther than this.

Hold for 1 minute in the beginning and gradually add seconds until 5 minutes are reached. Be accurate in your timing.

4. The most graceful way to come out of the posture is as follows: Bend your knees and lower them toward your forehead. Place the palms on the floor. Arch your neck upward (to keep the back of the head on the floor). Roll forward gracefully and with control. When your hips touch the floor straighten your legs into the position of Fig. 1. Slowly lower your legs to the floor and relax completely for 1 minute.

B-1

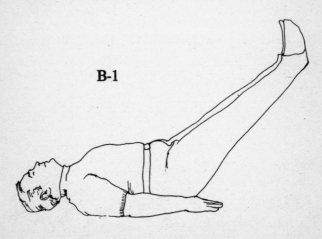

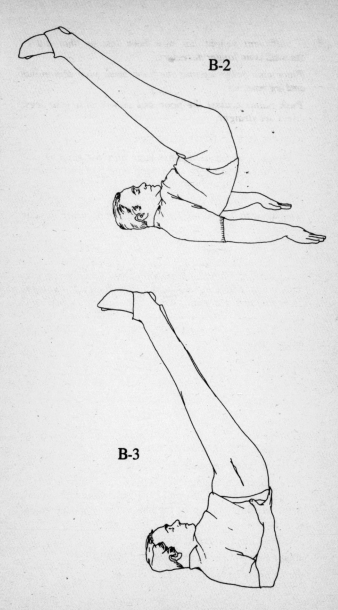

B-2

B-3

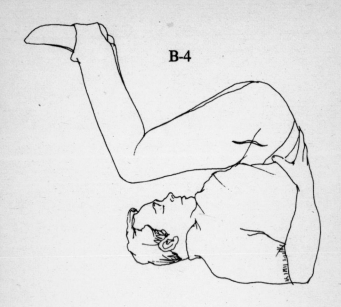

B-4

(C) Continued loss of weight will make this extreme position possible and highly effective.

Perform the movements of (B) 1-3.

Now slowly straighten your trunk and legs into this completely vertical position. The chin should be pressed firmly against the top of the chest. The body is straight but relaxed.

Hold for 3 to 5 minutes.

Come out of the posture as directed in (B) 4.

Relax in the lying position for 1 minute.

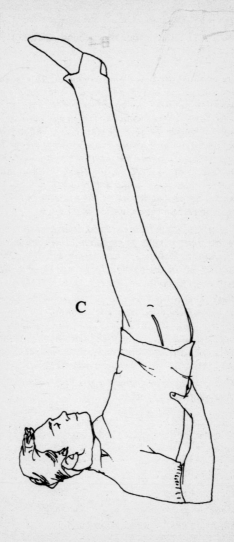

C

DEEP RELAXATION

(To attain a state of profound quietude)

(A) Lie as illustrated, allowing your body to rest in its most natural, comfortable position. Close your eyes. Place your consciousness on your feet and become very aware of your toes. Very gradually draw your consciousness upward through the feet, ankles, calves, knees, thighs and so on. As you become acutely aware of each of these areas, issue a gentle but firm order to all of the muscles in that area to "relax completely." Continue to draw the consciousness upward through the torso and neck, becoming acutely aware of the muscles in each area and making certain that none are held tensed

When you reach the neck area, transfer the consciousness to the tips of your fingers and slowly become aware of the hands, forearms, upper arms and shoulders. Again, you let go of all tension in each area and permit it to give in to the floor.

Next, concentrate on the face so that even these muscles are completely relaxed. At this point your entire organism will be in a state of deep relaxation. Spend two minutes or longer in this serene state and, in addition, attempt to "turn off" your mind so that no thoughts arise for this short period of time.

This exercise, performed correctly, is often equivalent to several hours of sleep.

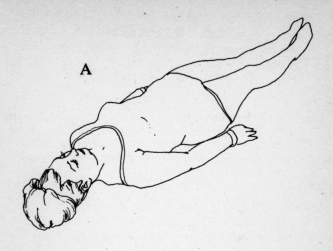

A

(B) & (C) The technique is identical with that of (A).

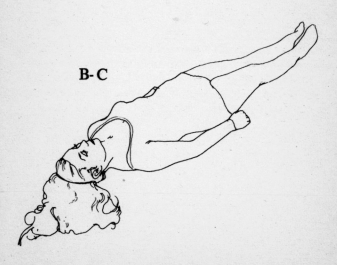

B-C

Perform 10 times

SECTION FOUR

YOGA
NUTRITION
MENUS

THE YOGA FOOD REGIMEN

The menus presented in this section are prototypes of the meals suggested for all serious students of Yoga. They are designed to accelerate weight loss and to permanently maintain your correct weight, once achieved.

The Yoga food regimen differs radically in concept from that of most "diets." To begin with, the word "diet" is a loser. One who is told that he has to "diet" is at an immediate psychological disadvantage; he knows full well the many denials and restrictions that are implicit. And regardless of how palatable the diet is made to appear ("eat pie for dessert once a day"; "pour this liquid appetite deterrent into a bowl and pretend it's soup"), the overweight person who has been accustomed to wielding a free knife and fork reacts with formidable negativity to the thought of self-imposed restrictions at mealtime. As long as the dieter feels that he is being denied the foods he really craves, as long as *restriction* is the keynote of the campaign, the battle is an uphill one.

For many years I have been observing people undertake various diets and the following pattern is the one which most often emerges: The dieter experiences a continual conflict between what he is allowed and what he really wants. Sooner or later he submits to his temptations and breaks the diet; this is followed, of course, by guilt, and a few more unsuccessful attempts are made, each with a little less resolve and a little more guilt and frustration. Eventually the diet is abandoned and this is followed by a great deal of guilt and usually a goodly number of pounds. In time, his weight condition will force him to go in search of another "miracle diet" and he will usually look for one in which the *restrictions* are more tolerable. Of the millions of Americans who each year undertake a diet, the percentage who remain on that diet for more than six months must be exceedingly low.

If a food regimen is to be truly effective it cannot be one that is undertaken for a few torturous weeks or months; it must not only impart the desired results but *must feel sufficiently natural and comfortable to become a way of life, to become permanent.* There can be no continually disquieting thoughts of being deprived or restricted. Therefore, imagine how pleasant it would be to shed excess pounds and inches if your organism *automatically* began to terminate those eating habits that add weight; that is, if you were *naturally* repelled by foods that are not only fattening but actually detract from the true joy of living! This is exactly the theory of Yoga nutrition. In what may be termed a "positive" approach, it suggests to the overweight person that, in accordance with several very basic principles, he is free to select whatever he desires from a great multitude of high-quality foods which will not add excess weight and which, in conjunction with his practice of the Yoga postures and breathing exercises, will sustain his organism in such an elevated state that he will find it virtually impossible to revert to his former eating habits.

Gradually he realizes that he is no longer in a battle, craving certain foods but being forced to adhere to an unnatural "diet"; something far more effective than will-power or guilt now prevails: *He simply loses his taste for what is harmful and fattening.* His body, functioning in a newly attained state of exhilaration, will not permit him to indulge in foods (or in any activity) that will alter this state and the wondrous part is that his organism can now *instinctively* avert those foods which are the offenders! How and why does this happen?

The body has a great innate wisdom, a universal intelligence that is in each of us and that is always ready to guide us in our true requirements, physical, emotional and spiritual. But because of our general living habits this wisdom often remains buried and either we do not hear the voice of guidance or we hear it very faintly. We turn to every conceivable *external* source to learn about ourselves when the truth of the matter is that the most authoritative information lies within. If you practice your Yoga physical and breathing exercises as directed in this book, you will quickly begin to experience what might be called a "liberation of the body." You will lose pounds and inches and, of course, feel lighter and more alive in all respects.

In freeing you of many physical as well as psychological encumbrances, Yoga also activates a great amount of life-force (prana) that is latent, sleeping within the organism. As this force is utilized there will be an acute sense of "getting with yourself"; you become increasingly attuned to the inner voice of wisdom and this voice serves as a most profound guide. You find yourself listening more and more with an inner ear to what your organism is saying, to its true requirements. And when you begin to act from this "center" of your being, you do so with an unshakable conviction of being *right*. Reliance on external sources in an effort to determine correct courses of action rapidly diminishes. This "direction" emanating from within is applied to all aspects of your life, including the establishment of the most beneficial eating habits.

Just as the practice of the Yoga exercises is designed to help eliminate negative patterns of the body and the meditation techniques are designed to liberate the mind, so will adherence to the principles of Yoga nutrition eventually free the student from those eating habits which not only result in excess weight but, equally important, decrease life-force and inhibit the body in functioning at that high level we wish to attain.

It must now be obvious that a paramount consideration of Yoga is that of acquiring and utilizing life-force. It becomes axiomatic that: the more life-force present in the organism, the higher the quality of life. Air, water and food are major sources of life-force. For this reason the serious student of Yoga will seek pure air (unpolluted), pure water (without chemical additives) and pure food. In connection with food, the word "pure" is synonymous with "natural." Foods that are consumed as close as possible to their natural state contain great quantities of life-force. To the extent that foods are denatured, that is, refined, canned, preserved, frozen, seasoned, smoked, aged, colored, fumigated, "enriched" and subjected to various processing, as well as cooked through such methods as roasting, boiling, frying, they are devitalized, rendered lifeless from our viewpoint.

You can fill your stomach with these substances and, if you have grown sufficiently desensitized, feel "satisfied" but, according to Yoga Nutrition, the true elements of nourishment, of life-force, are not present. For example, the fact that you do not immediately drop dead after finishing a typical seven-course restaurant dinner does not necessarily mean that you are receiving genuine nourishment from that meal. It is, rather, a testimonial to the remarkable strength of the organism, to how much abuse it can take day after day, year after year and still survive. But "survival" is not comparable to existing in the elevated state of which we have spoken.

The crux of the matter is: What you eat can either impart great life-force, vitality, energy, help regenerate your organism, regulate your weight and have a profoundly positive effect on your mind and emotions, or can sap your life-force, add excess weight, cause premature aging, be a contributing factor in many

181

illnesses and greatly lower the vibrations of the entire organism. Therefore, in determining what he will eat, the Yogi is not concerned with calories or with the idea of substitutions ("substitute margarine for butter, a chemical sweetener for refined sugar, lean meat for fat meat"), rather, he selects his foods from the standpoint of life-force, choosing those which are as close to their natural state as digestion permits and which will leave him feeling light and revitalized. Here is a remarkable fact for your consideration: *It is unnecessary to develop a weight-regulation program apart from or as a special aspect of Yoga Nutrition. With very few exceptions, one who follows the principles of Yoga Nutrition cannot help but attain and maintain his correct weight!*

The above ideas have been introduced as a preface to our menus. It is hoped that the reader will gain some insight into the fact that Yoga Nutrition offers a completely different approach not only to the weight problem but to the entire concept of what constitutes true nourishment; that it proposes a way of eating which, far from denying the student the "good" things of life, is designed to have him *experience* a level of well-being that is generally impossible to envisage. This book is meant to serve primarily as Yogic guidance in weight loss and control, and to achieve these objectives the student need not be fully versed in all of the details of Yoga Nutrition. If he will seriously undertake the menus of this section in conjunction with the Yoga exercise plan, the following can be accomplished:

(1) Loss of whatever excess weight is necessary.

(2) Maintenance of correct weight on a permanent basis.

(3) Eventual elimination of any sense of restriction or denial with regard to intelligent, healthful eating.

(4) Awakening of dormant life-force that enables "tuning in," becoming sensitive to the more *real* requirements of the entire organism.

(5) A raising of the organism's "vibrations," resulting in an unparalleled sense of well-being, optimism and awareness.

USING THE MENUS

The following pages contain two types of menus, labeled "Transition" and "Maintenance." There are two full weeks of menus offered for each type. The Transition Menus are to be followed during the first four weeks of the weight-loss program. Thereafter, the Maintenance Menus are utilized to complete and maintain the loss.

Without being extreme, the Transition menus introduce those foods and methods of preparation which we have been discussing. Within the eight-week period you will, to a great extent, "taper off" heavy flesh foods, starches, sugars, artificial stimulants and other substances on which you have been "hooked" these many years. Also, your taste buds will be purified and refined. You will then be ready to move into the Maintenance menus which are representative of the type of nutrition that should become a permanent part of your life.

Most of the foods and ingredients listed in the menus can be obtained from your usual shopping sources. However, in the light of this discussion you may be moved to search out those markets that offer the widest selection of truly fresh fruits and vegetables perhaps some *organic* produce (fruits and vegetables grown without the use of chemical fertilizers and sprays), more whole grain breads, possibly raw milk, very low-fat dairy products and unrefined sugar and flour products. If you have access to a health food store, become familiar with the items available, such as completely whole grain breads, unsulphured dried fruits, herb teas, cereal beverages, poly-unsaturated cooking and salad oils, fresh fruit and vegetable juices, raw nuts, etc.

If it is impossible for you to procure certain of the foods listed in our menus, it should be a simple matter to make intelligent substitutions once you are familiar with the "natural food" concept that underlies this entire program. Indeed, it is actually the intention of the author that these menus serve as *examples* of the types of foods, together with their combinations and preparations, that comprise Yoga Nutrition. This is especially true with regard to the Maintenance menus in which two weeks of meals cannot be expected to serve for a lifetime. However, we must reiterate that this book is primarily a guide for weight loss and you need not make any substitutions or devise any meals of your own unless you wish to do so. Simply following the given menus will enable you to achieve your objective.

You will, of course, notice the very limited listings of meat, coffee, dressings, condiments ·and other "staples" which are freely included in most so-called "reducing diets" and without which you may think that an agonizing death is imminent. But these omissions have been carefully calculated and are necessary in order that you may experience the dramatic changes we have discussed. Far from dying, you will be delighted to find that in direct proportion to the elimination of these negative substances you feel light, healthy, energized and "alive." (In passing it is worthwhile to note that many Yoga students who have followed our menus have lost their taste for nicotine and, as a consequence, have painlessly terminated the smoking habit!) It is possible that, in the initial stages of the Transition program, you will feel deprived with regard to certain foods, but you must remember that this occurs in the brain and the taste buds, not in the stomach. All such feelings of deprivation usually pass permanently within the course of a few weeks as you become more and more aware of the loss of weight and other positive changes that manifest themselves.

You must never become a bore or appear as a fanatic in your Yoga Nutrition program. It is best to be quiet and inoffensive about your activities along these lines. If you ever refuse to eat certain foods when you are out to dinner or at a social function, do so with a graceful excuse and do not make an issue of your refusal. Never tell another person that the foods which he or she is eating are harmful; you will be branded as a "food faddist," a "health nut," etc. We do not wish to force our ideas upon anyone. However, people are certain to notice the change in your physical appearance as well as *feel* the increased life-force radiating from you. A typical question will be, "You're looking wonderful. What have you been doing?" If you wish, you may mention one or two points about the program. If you meet with any scoffing or rejection, quietly drop the entire matter. But if someone appears to be sincerely interested and wants to know more, you may take them into your confidence. We attempt to conserve our life-force at all times and never to disperse it by becoming involved in useless argument or debate.

If you are the cook for your family, certain obstacles may arise. In many cases the family has gone right along with the student in both the Transition and Maintenance Menus. In these cases not only do the members of the family usually experience the same healthful benefits but, obviously, the problems for the student are minimized. However, if there are objections, you may have to prepare one type of meal for your family and another for yourself. All such extra efforts will be very much worth your while.

If you are under the care of a physician, consult him before undertaking any part of the Yoga Nutrition program.

186

NOTES ABOUT FOODS ON THE MENUS

Cooking methods: Steaming, baking and broiling are the best methods of cooking for our purposes. Avoid frying or using any substance that produces grease in cooking. Never boil or overcook your foods, especially vegetables. Heat them only until tenderized. Overcooking destroys life-force. Vegetables should always retain some crispness and not be soggy. Save and use as a broth or stock all of the juice produced from the cooking of vegetables.

Fruits and vegetables: Fresh fruits and fresh vegetables are always our first choice. Frozen products are a second choice when fresh produce is unavailable. We believe that canned fruits and vegetables contain very little life-force, being preserved with syrups, salt and chemical additives. Most fruits and many vegetables can and should be eaten raw, including the skins whenever possible. If your digestion will not permit raw foods, then stew or bake them lightly as indicated in the menus.

Dried fruits: Prunes, apricots, raisins, dates provide pure sugar energy and can be eaten in small quantities if between-meal snacks are an absolute necessity. They can also be soaked overnight for easy digestion. Read the label on the package in an attempt to obtain *unsulphured* products.

Dairy products: Our menus suggest the use of raw or non-fat milk, no cream or butter. Yogurt is indicated frequently; the most desirable type is *plain.* No flavored or fruit syrup yogurt should be consumed.

Cheeses: Dry or very lightly creamed cottage, farmer, ricotta, natural cheddar, Jack, genuine Swiss.

Sugars: In order of their desirability molasses (very high in iron), honey (obtain that which is uncooked, unbleached, unfiltered), raw sugar (unrefined), carob (ground St. John's bread; an excellent sweetening agent in powder form that can be utilized for many purposes). All fresh and dried fruits are high in natural sugar content. Refined sugar and artificial, chemical, "low-calorie" sweetening agents are never to be used.

Beverages: We urge the total elimination of coffee (caffeine is a drug) and teas that contain tannic acid. Herb teas and cereal beverages are suitable as after-meal drinks, if desired.

Seasonings: Vegetable salt and all edible herbs. Table salt, vinegar, prepared mustard; catsup and all hot spices should be eliminated.

Meat, poultry, fish: As indicated. For reasons that will be enumerated in subsequent writings, only calves' liver (an organ meat) is used in these menus. Broiled chicken livers are also indicated along with chicken and certain fish in the Transition Menus. No flesh food is used in the Maintenance Menus.

Whole grains: Only whole grain (no refined) products are desirable. Unrefined wheat, soya, bran, oats, millet, rye, barley can be used for cereals, breads and cakes. Date and banana breads and cakes, bran and soya muffins, rye crackers, etc. are all acceptable starches and are used in our menus.

Juices: Pure fruit and vegetable juices can be had at home with the use of a juicer and vegetable extractor. Most health food stores carry an assortment of natural juices. Canned and frozen juices that contain sugar and chemical additives should not be used.

Nuts: Unroasted and unsalted pecans, walnuts, cashews and almonds are suggested in small amounts. Most nuts are high in protein. (Peanuts are not suggested; the peanut is a legume.)

Nut butters: Become familiar with unsalted cashew and almond butters; these are delicious foods, very high in protein and superior to peanut butter. Consume in small quantities.

Eggs: If possible, obtain *fertilized* eggs. They contain all of the life-elements.

Sprouts: Fresh mung bean and alfalfa sprouts are delicious and high in mineral content. Available in most larger markets.

Oils: Poly-unsaturated oils should be used for cooking and dressings. Safflower, sesame and pure olive are suitable.

Dressings: Use the oils listed above, lemon juice and herbs.

Wheat germ: A concentrated source of protein, iron and vitamin E. Used in these menus as a natural supplement.

Brewers yeast: A basic source for the vitamin B group. Used in these menus as a natural supplement.

In the event that any of the lunches listed are impractical for those who work and must eat in restaurants or who do not have proper facilities to store the indicated foods, simply substitute those lunches that present no problem.

All recipes are for one serving. If additional servings are desired, increase the amounts accordingly.

Many of our recipes call for the use of a blender.

This appliance, and a vegetable juice extractor, are excellent investments in health.

Health food stores carry many natural foods indicated in our menus. A number of them now offer produce (fruits, vegetables) that has not been fumigated with chemical sprays.

TRANSITION MENUS

(To be used during the first
weeks of the regular program)

Note: If you undertake and complete the one week Partial Fast, these menus are to be used for the following three weeks. If you complete the one-week Liquid or Total Fast, bypass these menus and go directly to the Maintenance Menus.

1.   2.

Breakfast

Small bowl of dried fruit
(figs, prunes, apricots,
raisins, etc.), soaked
overnight if possible

Small bowl of cooked whole-
grain cereal; pure honey or
molasses; non-fat milk or
yogurt

Beverage (see "Notes")

Orange juice (freshly
squeezed if possible)

2 scrambled eggs (use
polyunsaturated margarine
for preparing)

Rye toast (1 slice) with
unsweetened peach or apple
butter

Lunch

Fruit salad
  Grapes, peaches, pineapple, pears with honey-yogurt
topping

Whole wheat crackers with
  cream cheese

Pineapple-Carrot Drink
  1/2 cup pineapple juice
  1/2 cup carrot juice
  1 tsp. lemon
  1 tsp. shredded coconut
  1 tsp. brewers yeast
  Blend
Whole-grain muffin

Dinner

Casserole
  Chicken baked with mushrooms, carrots, onions and
tomatoes

Sliced raw apple with na-
tural cheddar cheese

Salad
Crisp iceberg lettuce with
dressing made from 1/4 cup
cottage cheese, 1 tbsp. bleu
cheese and 1/4 cup yogurt.

Blend.

Fish chowder (bass and/or
halibut and/or sole)

Yogurt topped with sauce
made from fresh berries and
honey, whipped in blender

3.   4.

Breakfast

Small glass of pure grape juice

Honey-Cinnamon toast
  1/4 cup margarine
  1/4 cup honey

Blend. Spread on whole-grain bread. Sprinkle with cinnamon. Heat in broiler

Pineapple Drink
  1 cup pure pineapple juice
  1 tsp. parsley
  3 lettuce leaves
  1 tbsp. lemon juice

Blend

Whole-grain muffin

Lunch

Sliced avocado and tomato salad with lemon, safflower oil dressing

Whole wheat crackers

Tomato juice with lemon

1 slice pumpernickel (or other whole-grain bread) with cream cheese and alfalfa sprout spread

Dinner

Salad
  Napa cabbage, watercress, bermuda onion. Dressing: lemon juice and olive oil

Casserole
  Mushrooms and brown rice

Fresh papaya

Salad
  Sliced tomatoes with basil

Cheese souffle (natural cheddar)

Fruit compote

5.   6.

Breakfast

1/2 grapefruit

Large bowl of peaches and bananas; top with wheat germ and yogurt

Date-Nut Drink
  1 cup raw or non-fat milk
  1/2 cup pitted dates
  1 tbsp. nut butter
  1 tbsp. carob powder
    (optional)
Blend

Lunch

Coconut-Banana Drink
  1 banana
  1/2 cup coconut juice
  1 tbsp. wheat germ
  2 dates (pitted)
Blend
Bran muffin

Whole tomato stuffed with tuna salad

1 slice soya wheat toast with margarine

Dinner

Salad
  Romaine lettuce with parmesan cheese dressing
Whole wheat noodles with vegetarian tomato sauce
Honeydew melon

Salad
  Celery and carrot sticks
Soybeans stewed with tomatoes, onions
Pineapple chunks

Remember that you may fast as suggested!

Breakfast

Small glass grapefruit juice (freshly squeezed if possible)

Bowl of brown rice, raisins, honey or molasses, non-fat milk or yogurt

Banana Drink
1/4 cup pure orange juice
1 banana
pure vanilla
1 tbsp. honey
Blend

Lunch

Beet-Yogurt Drink
2 beets
1 cup tomato juice
1 tbsp. yogurt
1 tsp. parsley
Blend

Romaine lettuce salad with lemon-safflower oil dressing

Sesame seed crackers

Carrot-Date Salad
1/2 cup pitted dates
1 cup shredded carrots
1/2 cup chopped celery
1/4 cup yogurt
1/4 cup chopped nuts
Combine

Dinner

4 ozs. calves' liver (broiled and rare)

Salad of India
Sliced banana, 1/4 cup dates (pitted and chopped), sliced strawberries, mint sprinkled over top

Steamed fish (bass, halibut, sole)

Chinese vegetables:
Napa cabbage, snow peas, bean sprouts, mustard greens

Sherbet
Blend watermelon and sprig of mint. Freeze

9.   10.

Breakfast

Tomato juice (pure, if possible)

2-egg omelet (cooked in poly-unsaturated margarine)

1 slice whole-grain toast with margarine

1/2 cantaloupe filled with strawberries

Yogurt topping optional

Lunch

Orange-Yogurt Drink
  3/4 cup orange juice
  1/4 cup yogurt
  2 tbsp. honey
  pinch of mace or nutmeg

2 oatmeal cookies

Bowl of fresh vegetable soup

Whole-grain roll with margarine

Dinner

Salad
  Bibb lettuce and cherry tomatoes

Chicken livers (4) and brown rice (Livers broiled and rare)

Coconut custard

Escarole soup (chicken broth with escarole)

Egg foo yung

Honey-baked rhubarb

11.   12.

Breakfast

Swiss Breakfast
  1/4 cup rolled oatmeal
  1/4 cup yogurt
  1 tbsp. honey
  1/8 cup nuts, ground
  juice of 1/2 lemon
  1 apple, shredded

Combine. Non-fat milk may
be used if additional liquid is
desired.

Large slice of melon

Date-nut bread with cream
cheese (1 slice only)

Lunch

Apple juice

Nut butter mixed with raisins and spread on 1 slice of
whole-grain bread

Waldorf salad (substitute
yogurt for mayonnaise)

Whole wheat creackers

Dinner

Salad
  Cucumbers with lemon
juice

5 ozs. broiled halibut steak

Baked potato with margarine
and vegetable salt

Bowl of cherries

Salad
  Bell pepper, sliced, raw

Approximately 3/4 inch slice
of baked eggplant with ricotta cheese and tomato sauce

Fruit gelatin made with fresh
orange juice

13.   14.

Breakfast

Orange juice

Large bowl of strawberries and/or peaches topped with honey, yogurt and wheat germ

Small glass pure apple juice

2 buckwheat cakes with molasses or honey or pure maple syrup (no butter)

Lunch

Grape juice

Sandwich
 2 thin slices whole-grain bread (oatmeal, cracked-wheat, soya make excellent sandwich bread) with lettuce, tomato and cheddar cheese

Banana-Milk Drink
 1 banana
 1/2 cup raw or non-fat milk
 pinch of nutmeg

2 whole-grain cookies

Dinner

Egg-drop soup

2 whole tomatoes baked in olive oil and lemon juice

Brown rice pudding with cinnamon

Salad
 Romaine lettuce with chopped black olives

Chicken cacciatore

Bunch of cold grapes

MAINTENANCE MENUS

For permanent use, beginning the fifth week of the regular program

(If you complete the one week Liquid or Total Fast, these menus are for permanent use beginning the second week of the program.)

1.   2.

Breakfast

Banana Drink
  1 banana
  5 strawberries
  1/2 cup yogurt
Blend

Swiss Breakfast
  1/4 cup whole raw oats
  (soaked overnight if possible)
  2 apples, shredded
  1 tbsp. yogurt
  1 tbsp. honey
  1 tsp. lemon

Combine. Non-fat milk or
orange juice may be used if
additional liquid is desired

Lunch

Tomato juice

Chopped avocado and to-
mato salad on 1 slice whole-
grain bread

Bowl of fresh vegetables
(raw or lightly steamed)

Whole wheat crackers

Dinner

One baked bell pepper
stuffed with brown rice

Sliced peaches with cheddar
cheese

Salad
  1/4 cup young peas (raw)
  1/4 cup steamed string
  beans
  1/4 cup steamed aspara-
  gus tips

Moisten with French dressing

Mushrooms and onions sau-
teed

Honey-baked pears

3.   4.

Breakfast

Apple Drink
   1 cup pure apple juice
   1 tbsp. yogurt
   1 tsp. brewers yeast
Blend
1/2 cup mixed cashews/
raisins

Large bowl of fruit
   Strawberries/melon balls/
   peach slices
Yogurt topping optional

Lunch

Tomato stuffed with cottage
cheese and chives
Sesame crackers

Vegetable Drink
   1/3 cup beet juice
   1/3 cup carrot juice
   1 tbsp. brewers yeast
Blend
Several slices of mixed
cheeses: cheddar, Swiss,
jack; whole wheat crackers

Dinner

Raw vegetable dish
   Broccoli, tomatoes,
green peppers, Bermuda
onion (chopped), tossed
with yogurt
Brown rice pudding

Pure tomato soup
   Steam 3 tomatoes; blend
in blender; add vegetable salt
to taste
Zucchini, grated and baked.
Dot with margarine and
sprinkle with parmesan
cheese
Chunks of pineapple with
yogurt

5.   6.

Breakfast

Pineapple-Carrot Drink
  1/2 cup pineapple juice
  1/2 cup carrot juice
  1 tsp. lemon juice
  1 tsp. shredded coconut
  2 tsp. brewers yeast
Blend

Grape juice
1 slice whole-grain toast with nut-butter spread

Lunch

Apple juice
Cream cheese on one slice of date or banana bread

Salad
  Romaine lettuce
  1/2 cucumber
  1/2 green pepper
  1 stalk celery
  3 black olives

Slice, chop, combine

Dressing: tomato juice, safflower oil, lemon juice. Mix

1 slice rye toast

Dinner

Bowl of lentil soup (meatless)
Whole wheat crackers
Apple/carrot/orange salad

1/2 eggplant stuffed with sauteed onions and tomatoes and baked

Fruit cup
  Diced orange, sliced apricots, strawberries, 1/2 banana. Chill

7.   8.

Breakfast

Energy Drink
  1/2 cup prune or fig juice
  1/2 cup apple juice
  1 tsp. nut butter
  1 tsp. yogurt
  1 tsp. sesame or safflower oil
Blend

Large bowl of fruit
  cherries/watermelon,
  grapes/banana
Yogurt topping optional

Lunch

Vegetable-Cheese Salad
  Stalks of raw celery, carrot, broccoli, thin slices of cucumber, turnip, cheddar cheese
Whole wheat crackers

Potassium Drink
  1/4 cup carrot juice
  1/4 cup celery juice
  1/4 cup parsley juice
  1/4 cup watercress juice
Blend
Whole grain bread with slice of jack cheese

Dinner

Grapefruit and orange sections on lettuce
Steamed globe artichoke served with melted margarine
Banana cake

Casserole
  Zucchini, tomatoes, onion, natural cheese
Fruit compote

9.   10.

Breakfast

Date Milk
  1 cup non-fat or raw milk
  3 pitted, chopped dates
  1 tbsp. shredded coconut
  1 tsp. wheat germ
  1 tsp. safflower oil
Blend

Fresh orange juice
1 whole grain muffin
with apple butter spread

Lunch

Fruit Salad
  Sliced pineapple, peaches, pears with scoop of cottage cheese on bed of lettuce

Oatmeal cookies

1/2 avocado with olive oil and lemon
Wheat crackers

Dinner

Bowl of split-pea soup (meatless)

Apple dessert
  Apple slices sprinkled with sesame seeds, cinnamon, honey and lemon juice.
Bake

Salad
  Romaine lettuce, alfalfa sprouts. Dressing: olive oil and lemon juice

Welsh rarebit made with natural cheddar cheese; served over 1 slice whole-grain toast

Slice of watermelon

11.   ## 12.

Breakfast

Plum or papaya juice

Small bowl of cooked whole-grain cereal; 1 tsp. of honey or molasses; non-fat milk or yogurt

1/2 cantaloupe

1 slice date-nut bread with cream cheese spread

Lunch

Bowl of berries in season with 1/2 carton yogurt

Bran muffin

Bowl of tomato-brown rice soup

Sesame crackers with margarine or ricotta cheese

Dinner

Salad
    Cucumber and tomato slices

Watercress soup
    1/2 bunch watercress
    1 cup vegetable stock
    1/2 tsp. soy flour
    1/2 cup yogurt

Blend. (May be served hot or cold)

Wheat-germ raisin muffin

1/2 acorn squash, stuffed with:
    1/4 cup dried apricots
    1 tbsp. wheat germ
    1/3 cup whole grain bread crumbs
    1/4 cup hot cider

Blend and stuff into cavity of squash. Bake.

Honeydew melon

13.   14.

Breakfast

Large bowl of fruit
  sliced oranges
  sliced apples
  raisins
  yogurt topping

1/2 grapefruit

Soy flour (or whole-wheat flour) waffle, molasses or pure maple syrup

Lunch

Slice of melon

Dates and nuts chopped and mixed into cream cheese; spread on one slice of whole-grain bread

Pineapple-Carrot Drink
  1/2 cup pineapple juice
  1/2 cup carrot juice
  1 tsp. lemon
  1 tsp. shredded coconut
  1 tsp. brewers yeast
Blend

Dinner

Salad
  Raw mung bean sprouts with French dressing

Bowl of black bean soup

Soya muffin

Brown rice and herbs with mushrooms

Raw apple-sauce

MAINTENANCE

Having accomplished your goal, you can now maintain your correct weight by faithfully performing the exercises of C, continuing to apply the principles of nutrition as outlined in the menus and by incorporating as much as possible of the Yoga philosophy and meditation practice into your daily life.

YOGA FOR HEALTH
*Mr. Hittleman's TV series can
be seen in many areas.
You may correspond with him personally
regarding this weight loss
program by writing to:
Richard Hittleman,
P.O. Box 554
Santa Cruz, California
95061*